TUTORIALS IN
GENERAL PRACTICE

To our wives, Elaine and Beryl

For Churchill Livingstone:

Commissioning Editor: Ellen Green
Project Editor: Janice Urquhart
Project Controller: Nancy Arnott
Design direction: Erik Bigland

TUTORIALS IN GENERAL PRACTICE

Michael Mead BSc MB DRCOG DCH MRCGP

Henry R. Patterson MA MD FRCGP DOBSTRCOG

THIRD EDITION

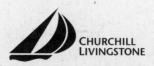
CHURCHILL
LIVINGSTONE

EDINBURGH LONDON NEW YORK OXFORD PHILADELPHIA ST LOUIS SYDNEY TORONTO 1999

CHURCHILL LIVINGSTONE
An imprint of Elsevier Science Limited

225480033

First published 1983
Second edition 1992
Third edition 1999
 Reprinted 2001, 2002, 2003

ISBN 0 443 06197 1

British Library Cataloguing in Publication Data
A catalogue record for this book is available from the British
Library.

Library of Congress Cataloging in Publication Data
A catalog record for this book is available from the Library of
Congress.

Medical knowledge is constantly changing. As new information
becomes available, changes in treatment, procedures, equipment
and the use of drugs become necessary. The authors and the
publishers have, as far as it is possible, taken care to ensure that
the information given in this text is accurate and up to date.
However, readers are strongly advised to confirm that the
information, especially with regard to drug usage, complies with
the latest legislation and standards of practice.

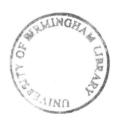

 your source for books,
journals and multimedia
in the health sciences
www.elsevierhealth.com

The
publisher's
policy is to use
**paper manufactured
from sustainable forests**

Printed in China
B/04

PREFACE TO THE THIRD EDITION

When we were approached to write a third edition of *Tutorials*, we were surprised. After all it was originally written as a trainer/registrar project. Surely it is getting rather dated? So we sat down and read it from cover to cover. To our surprise many of the issues and problems have hardly changed – for example, the principles of terminal care which we produced in the first edition have been followed by new modern 'guidelines' which have scarcely changed at all. This applies to many of the subjects.

The patients and their problems are the same now as they were when we started to write tutorials. What has changed is the knowledge available, new drugs and their effect on management, new health promotion strategies, and so on. To give one example, we thought that the chapter on croup was obsolete because we rarely see problems arising now due to respiratory obstruction, but this is for two very good reasons. Firstly, the introduction of Hib vaccination has reduced the incidence of acute epiglottitis, and, secondly, the use of a nebulizer containing steroids is effective.

This gave us our answer. There are new generations of registrars coming forward, facing the same problems as their predecessors but in the setting of a changed health service, the emergence of new treatments and considerable emphasis on evidence-based decisions. We have therefore reviewed all chapters in this light, adding where necessary new facts and treatments and drawing on published guidelines for management, which are clearly going to influence the delivery of care in the foreseeable future.

Medicine has advanced rapidly since the second edition of this book was published in 1992. In this third edition there has been a considerable updating of the text to keep the content relevant to medicine in the year 2000. There are new chapters on audit and project work, both of increasing importance to the doctor entering family practice in the future.

H.P. 1999
M.M.

FOREWORD TO THE FIRST EDITION

Much of the literature about teaching in general practice stresses the reciprocal nature of the teacher–learner relationship. Here is a book written by a general practitioner trainer and his registrar. The approach is practical, the conditions dealt with are those most commonly encountered in general practice, the style is brisk, and the tone, unusual for a book about general practice, is firmly didactic.

Much has been written about the deficiencies of medical education in preparing doctors for an imaginative use of the doctor–patient relationship, or for an understanding of the needs of practice populations and how they might be met. Much less is written about the absence of sound clinical training about those diseases which, by and large, are not presented in the hospital, are not life threatening but constitute a major source of distress. Many of us have the suspicion that what we know about in medicine are the very commonest conditions with which we deal.

This book should be welcomed by registrars and trainers in general practice alike. I predict that it will not only be used as a handbook on the registrar's desk, but that its chapters will form the basis of clinical tutorials and audits in teaching practices.

Marshall Marinker
Director, The MSD Foundation

PREFACE TO THE FIRST EDITION

'Teaching and learning in the period of postgraduate education are primarily concerned with the development of the specific skills and the acquisition of specific knowledge on which general practice depends. It is also concerned with the development of the trainee's critical faculties. Trainers need to recognize and define their students' individual strengths and weaknesses. There is no immutable curriculum.'

Marinker

This book is, we think, unique. It represents the results of a series of dialogues. Firstly, it is the debate between a trainer and a registrar in general practice, to find what the registrar needs to learn, what it is the trainer has to teach, and how this might be achieved. This discussion took place during the registrar's first and second year when he had a short 3-month introductory period in general practice and then returned to his hospital posts. The initial period in general practice highlighted the gaps in his knowledge and skills, of which he became acutely aware. This stimulated a search for appropriate literature, with disappointing results. We thus had to choose which tutorials should take place.

Some of these were registrar initiated: 'I need to know how to treat the acute ear in general practice.' Others were suggested by the trainer: 'You really should look more closely at your management of the hypertensive patient.'

The stimulus was that the subject was perceived by one of us to be important and we were guided in this by the clinical material which was passing through the practice at the time and the many excellent topic lists which are available.

We prepared some material and discussed it, then collected more relevant information and produced a written record of the tutorial.

We then decided that we were really writing a book which does not exist elsewhere; why not try to get it published? Thus our second dialogue was between ourselves and our publishers. They gave us the necessary impetus to carry the task through. We had to decide what was of interest to trainers and registrars in general and to those doctors who are training for general practice but have not joined a formal scheme. The constraints of a deadline were most valuable in this task.

Each chapter therefore contains an introductory paragraph giving basic information about the problem or symptom which can be obtained from a review of the literature, on the nature of the problem, its incidence and prevalence, and a comment on its significance. Next, there is a brief outline of a case as it is presented. The presentation is divided into steps and the tutorial discussion takes place as the problem unfolds. We were most careful to identify at this stage the factual knowledge which was required, and most of this is presented in tables or lists for easy reference. The tutorial emphasizes the history and examination thought to be relevant and discusses at length issues which were raised. Finally, where possible, the outcome of the case is recorded and a summary of the teaching points is given for any future revision. The addition of some multiple choice questions at the end of the book has been made so that the reader may test recall of the chapter.

Thirdly, the dialogue is between us and you, the reader. We have committed ourselves to paper and have said what we think is relevant, interesting and important. We hope that it will stimulate you and perhaps help you. Most of all we hope that it will challenge you to produce something better for yourselves.

We should like to thank Mrs Carol Coley for her help in typing the manuscript and Mr Chorley of the Audiovisual Department of Leicester University for drawing the illustrations; and finally our composite and heavily disguised patients, without whom there would have been no book.

M.M.   H.P.

CONTENTS

1 THE TUTORIAL

The tutorial is the kernel of the teaching programme during the training year in practice. It is a most powerful teaching tool. Each week the trainer and registrar agree to spend an uninterrupted period of time together for educational purposes. This is an unusual experience for both, for not only is the tutorial in general practice a relatively recent development, most doctors have never in the course of their long training had a period exclusively devoted to teaching by one person.

Certain questions form in the mind of any trainer faced with a new registrar. These usually take the form of 'What sort of registrar are you?', 'What do you know already?', 'What are my aims and what do you seek from me?', 'How do we decide what to do and how shall we set about doing it?' and finally, 'How do we know we have been successful in any given tutorial?'.

Becoming a registrar in general practice represents a culture shock. From the hospital world of precise diagnosis and intense investigation, the registrar is faced with a different world of grey areas, ill-defined symptoms and signs, and minor illnesses never previously mentioned at medical school. Hay fever, acne and coughs are now the order of the day, rather than Crohn's disease or sarcoidosis. Patients present with insoluble problems which have no basis in the structured format of traditional medical education. Patients come for tranquillizers after a divorce, break down and cry in the surgery, or become angry at the way life has treated them. Initially these consultations are very difficult for the registrar, and the opportunity of listening to an experienced general practitioner communicating to such patients is invaluable in providing a model on which the registrar can base his or her own consultation skills.

The development of a good relationship between a trainer and registrar is essential for tutorial work. There must be an openness of discussion, a frankness in explaining difficulties and a healthy criticism of approach. The tendency for tutorials to develop into a cosy chat must be strongly resisted. An informal 'hour over coffee' with a few political asides and a comment on the state of the local football team may be pleasant enough, but will not serve the registrar well in the long term. Tutorials must be structured and well prepared, with a precise remit and an evaluation of what has been achieved.

Giving a tutorial is an acquired art that needs to be learned. Each new registrar poses different problems for the trainer. The best tutorials are joint ventures and it may be difficult to define who is the learner and who the teacher. Tutorials can be just as stimulating for the trainer as for the registrar.

Aims of the tutorial

Ten aims of the tutorial are listed in Box 1.1. The main aim, undoubtedly, must be to motivate for the future, encouraging the registrar to develop an interest in general practice that will hopefully be lifelong. Among the other aims listed, providing the registrar with a sound clinical acumen relevant to general practice is of obvious importance. It is essential that all aspects of practice management are fully covered, to equip the registrar for coping with the day he or she becomes a partner.

How often?

There is evidence that registrars wish to have more tutorial time than they receive. A 2- to 3-hour weekly session is most valuable for a tutorial as it allows time to explore and enlarge any debate. As well as a formal tutorial, informal discussion should be encouraged, and not just with the named trainer. Similarly, the registrar should have 'sitting in' sessions with the other partners, thus widening his or her experience of the different approaches to a consultation.

Box 1.1 Aims of the tutorial

1. To stimulate interest in the subject being discussed and in general practice as a whole
2. To instil in the registrar a spirit of inquiry and to encourage problem-solving abilities
3. To instil in the registrar a sense of professional values
4. To formulate management plans for specific patients and for common conditions
5. To identify key problem areas for discussion and to direct the registrar to sources of further information
6. To help the registrar develop his or her consultation skills
7. To help the registrar develop an understanding of how patients behave, why they consult, what they expect, etc.
8. To explain the principles of practice management
9. To encourage a critical and sensible attitude to prescribing
10. By means of a syllabus of tutorials:
    a. to help prepare the registrar for a future partnership
    b. to help prepare the registrar for the MRCGP examination
    c. to provide a sound clinical basis for patient management

Content

Some sort of check-list must be made. There will be a changing need over the 3 years of the training period.

In the first year the need will be for training in the common clinical conditions a general practitioner encounters. Prominent here will be the management of patients with sore throats, hay fever, earache, acne, cystitis and similar topics.

In the middle year the registrar should be exploring the protocols for managing chronic conditions like asthma or diabetes. Prescribing will be a key area, as will confidentiality and ethics. Some of the more difficult consultations should be covered here—a patient who is 'tired all the time' for example.

In the third and last year, with the prospect of a partnership looming, practice management will need to be covered in depth. Ideally, in forming the syllabus, there should be a mixture of trainer-initiated tutorials ('You should look at your prescribing of antibiotics.') and registrar-initiated tutorials ('I'd like to know more about how a practice employs its staff.').

A trainer should not underestimate the registrar Many have a great deal of factual knowledge and have gained considerable experience in dealing with medical emergencies while in hospital. A tutorial on chest infections should therefore concentrate on the difficulties special to general practice rather than differential medical diagnoses—how you would manage an 80-year-old lady with a chest infection at home, for example.

There are four main areas that are the key to a successful tutorial.

1. Relevance
Unless the topic is seen to be relevant to the registrar, no matter how interesting it is to the trainer, the tutorial will fail. For example, an interesting presentation on the choice of a practice will hardly be well received when given to a registrar in the first 3 months, but may be a resounding success in the final year.

2. Sequence
Topics covered must be tackled in the correct sequence. It is difficult to appreciate the ethical considerations if a registrar is still worried about the mechanics of referring someone for a termination of pregnancy.

3. Active involvement
An adult learns as much by doing as by listening. The registrar should be involved in the tutorial, not only in discussion but in some preparation and follow-up. This is why using clinical material from previous surgeries is valuable. He or she remains a resource as well as a participant and this guarantees relevance.

4. Information about performance
A criticism often voiced by registrars is that they do not know how they are getting on, and that when problems arise they are unaware that these were even detected by their trainer. The trainer should develop the habit of feeding information back to the registrar about his or her clinical performance, balancing praise with criticism.

Teaching techniques

Various teaching techniques can be used during a tutorial, for example:

- active involvement, e.g. role play
- audiovisual techniques
- patient management questionnaires
- multiple choice questions
- log diary sessions
- case discussions
- discussion of specific topics.

Conduct of the tutorial

A tutorial should take place in a relaxed environment with no possibility of an urgent visit to interrupt the flow! Preparation is important, so references should have been made available before-hand in case they are needed during the discussion. The registrar should ideally do much of the work—thoughts and ideas being channelled and directed by the trainer, with the aid of reference material.

A questioning rather than a didactic approach will usually reap the greatest dividends. This approach (outlined in Box 1.2) involves identifying a problem, which may have arisen from a particular consultation, and expanding the problem to raise wider issues. These issues are then discussed and gaps in knowledge identified. The trainer and registrar then attempt to fill these gaps by a literature search and come together finally for a follow-up to complete the tutorial. This follow-up stage is important and can form the start of the next tutorial. Education is a continuous process and a 'tutorial' never really ends; to some extent the whole of training is a tutorial.

Box 1.2   The questioning approach to a tutorial

Step 1   Questioning around a patient/case history e.g. Mrs Jones presents with cystitis:

   a. *Questions concerning the consultation*:
   Why did Mrs Jones attend when she did?
   What questions did you ask her?
   Why did you ask for an MSU?
   What general advice did you give?
   Did you prescribe?

   b. *Critical evaluation*:
   Why did/didn't you ask for an MSU?
   Why a 7-day rather than a 3- or 1-day course of antibiotics?
   Why did you choose trimethoprim?

Step 2   Identify a problem:
   How do we manage patients with cystitis?

Step 3   Expand the problem:
   How commonly do patients present with cystitis?
   What sort of patients present?
   Is it worth doing an MSU in every case?
   What is the best treatment?
   What about patients with recurrent cystitis?
   Are there any patients who should be referred?

Step 4   Discussion of viewpoints of registrar and trainer on these problems

Step 5   Identification of gaps in knowledge. Trainer and registrar to consult books, references, etc. to fill these gaps

Step 6   Follow-up. The gathering together of all the information and the formulation of a policy/management protocol on how to manage patients with cystitis

2 A SORE THROAT

Sore throat is the seventh most common symptom in primary care: 12% of adults and 8% of children reported this symptom in a sample 2-week period. The incidence can quadruple between summer and winter months. An average general practitioner in this country may expect to see about 250 cases a year. Sore throats are common up to the age of 45 and then decline slightly.

A boy, George Sandown, 16 years old, came to the surgery with his mother. 'He has a terrible sore throat,' she said anxiously. I could find little to support this. He was apyrexial, with slight enlargement of the tonsillar lymph glands. There was some redness of the tonsillar fauces extending up onto the soft palate.

What are the diagnostic possibilities?

CAUSES OF SORE THROAT

The majority of sore throats encountered will be of viral aetiology and will last for up to 4 or 5 days. The common viruses encountered are:

- herpes virus
- influenza virus
- enterovirus
- rhinovirus
- adenovirus.

Of the bacterial causes, β-haemolytic streptococci are the most important (Fig. 2.1). Streptococci are isolated from about a third of teenagers/adults, 50% of children aged 4–13 and only 15% of children under age 3 years. Others are:

- *Haemophilus influenzae*
- Staphylococci—which may be pathogenic or commensal
- *Streptococcus pneumoniae*.

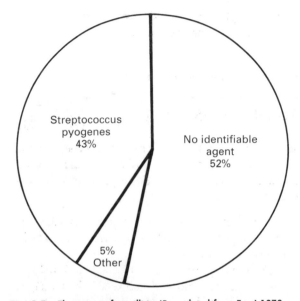

Fig. 2.1 The causes of tonsillitis. (Reproduced from Fry J 1979 *Common diseases, their nature, incidence and care.* MTP Press, by permission of author and publisher.)

Other rarer but important causes:

- Epstein–Barr virus (infectious mononucleosis)
- Monilia
- diphtheria
- Vincent's angina
- irritants, e.g. cigarette smoking
- blood dyscrasias
- neoplasm
- psychological factors
- pathogens from the genital tract.

The appearance of the tonsils and pharynx are not a reliable indication of the infecting organism. Typical features of a streptococcal sore throat are pain, fever of sudden onset, pain on swallowing. Tonsillar or pharyngeal exudate and enlarged anterior cervical lymph nodes support but do not prove a streptococcal aetiology. The probability is that this is a viral infection, self-limiting and not serious.

What other information should be sought?

1. The duration of the symptoms
2. Evidence of systemic upset, fever or other symptoms indicating the degree of illness
3. Past history
4. Social implications—family commitments, impending examinations, etc.

How do you decide on treatment?

TREATMENT OF SORE THROAT

The use of penicillin in the treatment of sore throat has been a contentious issue for many years. It is worth summarizing the position. The arguments in favour of prescribing penicillin are:

1. If a bacterial cause is present it is likely to respond to penicillin (although there is increasing resistance to penicillin).
2. The prescription of penicillin may have reduced the incidence of serious sequelae of β-haemolytic streptococcal infections, i.e. rheumatic fever and acute glomerulonephritis.
3. Taking a swab is impracticable—the availability of pathological laboratory facilities, the time scale involved and the relative cost all make it unlikely that the decision to treat can await the result of this test. Only a minority of viruses can be cultured even when a suitable transport medium is used. Rapid antigen tests are available now, having 90% specificity and sensitivity, but are still not a practical proposition for daily general practice.
4. A sore throat can be a relatively severe illness involving constitutional upset, pyrexia, vomiting, swollen glands and loss of time from work.
5. It has been said that penicillin reduces the duration of the illness by approximately 24 hours.
6. Penicillin is cheap and safe. Anaphylactic shock after the administration of penicillin is very rare. The incidence is about 0.02%. In one series of 793 cases of anaphylaxis following penicillin, only 49 were due to oral preparations. (*Source: Leicestershire Drug Information Service.*)

7. An antibiotic continued for 10 days will eliminate bacteria from the upper respiratory tract.

The arguments against prescribing penicillin are:

1. In most cases the treatment is ineffective.
2. The clinical appearance of the throat is no indication of its aetiology.
3. The reduction in the incidence of serious sequelae may be due to a change in the virulence of the streptococci and not to the use of penicillin.
4. Many streptococcal illnesses are not associated with symptoms.
5. There is a danger of producing penicillin-resistant organisms.
6. There is a danger of producing sensitivity to penicillin.
7. The side-effects of antibiotics include gastro-intestinal disease, rashes and vaginal candidiasis.
8. The prescription of an antibiotic educates the patient to expect similar treatment on a subsequent occasion.
9. Anaphylactic shock may be produced.

Published studies do not support the routine use of antibiotics for patients with a sore throat. Little et al (*BMJ* 1997; 315: 350–352) randomized patients aged 4 and over with sore throats to three groups: a 10-day prescription of antibiotics, no antibiotics, and a delayed prescription if the sore throat had not settled after 3 days. There was no difference between the groups in early return or complications but prescribing for sore throats encouraged reattendance for sore throat in the future. Giving a prescription increases the medicalization of a self-limiting illness.

There are therefore no grounds for a doctor to prescribe an antibiotic for a self-limiting upper respiratory tract infection. Doctors are likely to encounter difficulties in following this advice because:

1. Psychosocial factors are often involved in the decision to prescribe.
2. Belief in the prevention of complications is still held to be valid by many.
3. Patients have been educated to expect antibiotics.
4. Doctors are anxious to please their patients.
5. A consistent practice policy would be needed to curtail the use of antibiotics.
6. Doctors may save time in a consultation by issuing a prescription.

A pragmatic solution as to whether to prescribe or not would be to:

- prescribe in patients with a severe pharyngitis with pronounced systemic symptoms or in those with a scarlet fever rash
- to have a lower threshold for prescribing in children aged 4–13 who have a higher probability of a bacterial cause
- to have a lower threshold for prescribing if there is a streptococcal outbreak in the practice, the patient is a contact of a known case or is immunosuppressed.

Practices that have an antibiotic prescribing policy to which all adhere have a far better chance of re-educating their patients to accept that antibiotics have only a small part to play in the management of sore throat.

George had had a sore throat for 7 days. He had consulted a doctor for this symptom seven times in the past 2 years. Each time he had been prescribed penicillin, by different partners.

What diagnosis do you consider and how would you proceed?

INFECTIOUS MONONUCLEOSIS (GLANDULAR FEVER)

Probably the most common cause of sore throats that fail to resolve within 7 days is infectious mononucleosis (glandular fever). Its peak incidence occurs in teenagers and young adults. The hallmarks of this condition are:

1. clinical features
2. blood picture
3. serological findings.

Other diseases that can give a similar picture are:

1. toxoplasmosis
2. cytomegalic virus infection
3. infectious lymphocytosis
4. drug reaction.

The clinical features of glandular fever are shown in Box 2.1.

Box 2.1   Clinical features of infectious mononucleosis

Symptoms of glandular fever
1. Slow onset of malaise (1–6 weeks)
2. Vague symptoms including pyrexia, headache, myalgia and anorexia
3. Sore throat (85%), cervical adenitis (95%), rash (10%), rash if exposed to ampicillin (95%)
4. Dyspepsia

Clinical findings
1. Pharyngitis, petechial haemorrhages of the palate
2. Adenitis—cervical, axillary, groins
3. Rash—erythematous, urticarial, macular or papular after exposure to ampicillin
4. Splenomegaly (50%)
5. Jaundice +/– hepatomegaly (5–10%)

Blood picture

There is a characteristic abnormality of the white cells in which atypical mononuclear cells are found in increasing numbers. There is also a relative lymphocytosis. The serum contains antibodies to the red cells of some animals. These are known as heterophil antibodies.

The Epstein–Barr virus, which is now known to be the aetiological agent, affects the B lymphocytes. It is thought that these are stimulated when they are already committed to produce antibodies. This has been likened to blowing on a trumpet which gives an uncertain sound.

Serology

The heterophil antibodies can be detected, and this is the basis of the Paul–Bunnell test. The sensitivity has been improved by using guinea pig absorption techniques, and commercial methods such as the Monospot test are now used. All tests have similar specificity. Heterophil antibodies may persist for many months, even years. The presence of these antibodies may signify past infection and not necessarily a relapse.

Antibodies to the Epstein–Barr virus itself can now be detected by a fluorescent antibody staining technique. The antibodies appear early and the titre rises rapidly and may be missed. A single titre of the antibody against the Epstein–Barr virus of 1:80 or higher, or the presence of specific IgM, may be accepted as diagnostic.

Confirming the diagnosis

It should be remembered that no one test is infallible. The Monospot test remains a rapid and easily available means of diagnosis, although it may take 2–3 weeks to turn positive. Specific tests for antibodies for the Epstein–Barr virus should resolve most doubtful cases.

A throat swab is unlikely to be of value in this instance. It will be negative in the case of glandular fever, and 10% of the population carry β-haemolytic streptococci with or without symptoms. The result of this test is unlikely to influence your management. Swabs in viral transport medium have a low positive culture rate (30%).

A blood count should show the presence of atypical mononuclear cells and a lymphocytosis. A Paul–Bunnell or Monospot test is likely to be positive in 90% of cases (less in children). If the clinical picture is strongly suggestive and the Monospot test negative, tests for Epstein–Barr virus may resolve the issue.

Glandular fever, if diagnosed, usually runs an uncomplicated course over about 6–8 weeks, but sometimes the lassitude and malaise may be prolonged for periods of up to a year. Among the rare but possible complications are a ruptured spleen, respiratory obstruction, meningitis, peripheral neuritis, acute haemolytic anaemia, myocarditis, pericarditis, nephritis and nephrosis.

Management

1. There is no specific treatment
2. Rest during the acute stages
3. Aspirin gargle for sore throat
4. Steroids have been advocated in severe infections
5. Antibiotics for secondary infection (avoid amoxycillin).

TONSILLECTOMY

With George's recurrent history of sore throats, Mrs Sandown was probably thinking of tonsillectomy, and

this should be anticipated. There is only one absolute indication for tonsillectomy: peritonsillar abscess which has a tendency to recur and can produce serious respiratory obstruction. The MRC trial of tonsillectomy in the 5- to 7-year-old age group failed to demonstrate the advantages of the treated over the untreated group, and the question of whether tonsillectomy impairs the body's response to infection in the future has not been satisfactorily answered. The indications for operation are therefore a matter of debate, but the following would seem reasonable guidelines:

1. Recurrent tonsillitis sufficient to impair and interfere with the patient's normal life. This is taken to mean five attacks a year associated with malaise and a period of time off work or school.
2. Recurrent tonsillitis in a teenager or adult suggests persistently infected tonsillar tissue and is more readily accepted as an indication for tonsillectomy, although the operation itself is more hazardous.
3. Tonsillar hypertrophy of a size sufficient to cause sleep apnoea.
4. Unilateral tonsillar enlargement.

Parental expectations and the policy of long waiting lists for tonsillectomy generate a demand for private treatment. By the time the request has been made parents are usually unhappy with the situation and careful discussion is indicated, as it may mean there has been a failure in communication between the doctor and the family at an earlier stage.

A PLAN OF MANAGEMENT

In George's case a plan of management should be formed.

1. An examination specifically for the signs of glandular fever or other diseases should be made.
2. A full blood count, looking for the presence of atypical mononuclear cells and a relative lymphocytosis, with a request for the Monospot test for heterophil antibodies.
3. Some symptomatic treatment should be offered; a gargle such as aspirin would relieve his sore throat and help the accompanying malaise.
4. Preparatory discussion with his mother, explaining the reasons for tonsillectomy and offering a further

opinion if the condition does not resolve, or if there is a recurrence in the near future.

5. Ask Mrs Sandown and George for their views and whether they find the above suggestions acceptable.

If glandular fever is excluded and the condition continues to recur within the predicted period, it would be reasonable to seek an ENT consultant's opinion.

TEACHING POINTS

1. The appearance of a sore throat is no indication of its aetiology.
2. There is now no good argument for prescribing penicillin routinely.
3. Glandular fever should be considered.
4. Indications for tonsillectomy should act as a starting point for discussion.

3 ACNE AND WARTS

Skin conditions form 15% of all consultations in general practice. They are not life threatening and often the problem seems minimal to the general practitioner; but to the patient they can not only be irritant but socially embarrassing so that his or her way of life is altered. With a little care and attention on the part of the general practitioner and some persistence by the patient (as the treatment is often prolonged), these can be among the most satisfying conditions to treat. An immense range of skin conditions presents to the general practitioner, but the most common are listed in Table 3.1. Verrucae (plantar warts) alone are said to cause 60 consultations per 1000 patients aged 5–14 each year (Hart, *Child Care in General Practice*).

ACNE

Shaun Dickson, a shy and self-conscious boy of 17, came to the surgery to see if there was anything I could give him for his acne. He was very hesitant and it had obviously taken a lot of courage for him to present himself. He felt sure there was nothing I could do about his condition, but he had been persuaded to come 'just in case'. I saw that he had quite a few comedones on his cheeks and around his chin, with a few reddened papules on the right side of the chin. His back, or at least its upper part, was more severely affected, with large papular lesions and an occasional pustule. I assured him that there was treatment available.

Is this a typical case of acne?

Is Shaun's case typical in terms of:

1. age of the patient
2. distribution of the acne
3. the lesions present?

   1. Yes. Acne is really largely a disorder of adolescence. It begins at puberty but may appear just before; hence girls tend to develop the problem earlier than boys. Acne is an inflammatory process affecting the sebaceous glands and their associated hair follicles distributed over the face, arms, back and chest. Testosterone stimulates the sebaceous glands to produce sebum and oils which lubricate the skin. The glands are inactive in prepubertal children. Acne results from abnormal growth of the cells lining the duct from the gland to the outside of the skin. They stick to the inside of this canal, furring it up like the pipes in a central heating system. Once blocked, a plug of solidified sebum forms the easily recognized blackhead. The trapped liquid sebum is a food for the skin bacterium *Propionibacterium acnes* which stimulates the immune system and causes the inflammatory reaction that shows as redness around the spot. Eventually the gland may burst, sending its contents into the surrounding tissues. It is thought that 85% of adolescents will have some degree of acne but only a small proportion seek advice from a doctor. The peak incidence is about the 19th year, but very rarely it can start in the third and fourth decades of life. The natural history of the disease is a little unpredictable; in very mild forms it may only last

Table 3.1 Skin disease in general practice

Condition	Incidence (%)
Acute infection (including fungal infections)	33
Eczema	30
Warts	9
Urticaria	6
Pruritus	5
Acne	4
Psoriasis	3
Pityriasis rosea	1
Other	9

< 1% admitted to hospital
< 1% of all deaths due to skin disease
13% of the population consult with skin disease each year

a few months but it usually lasts until the early 20s, so that it would be reasonable to say to patients that in the majority of cases people have 'grown out of' their acne by 25. It is however impossible to predict an age for an individual patient—it can in fact persist until middle age.

2. Yes. Acne lesions occur on the face, back and chest—these areas having the largest number of sebaceous glands. The face is usually the worst affected and it may only occur in parts of the face. Occasionally the back is more severely affected and is nearly always more affected than the chest.

3. Yes. There are four main lesions of acne. The first is the blackhead or comedone—a keratin plug with retained thickened sebum. The second type is the papule, of varying degrees of redness depending on the inflammatory reaction around the follicular orifices; these may progress to pustules and finally to cysts. A comedone may disappear spontaneously without causing any inflammation. Acne may be followed by scarring—usually seen as a pitting. Keloid formation may occur. The lesions of acne may be found together or alone—in some cases there will only be papules and pustules while some will only have comedones. Picking and squeezing the lesions results in superficial sores and crusts. Premenstrual exacerbation is well recognized.

Many factors seem to be responsible for acne: an increased sebum excretion rate (promoted by androgens), an obliteration of the pilosebaceous canal, and bacterial involvement all seem to be important.

Is there a diet that may be useful?

No. There is a widespread belief that fatty or fried foods, sweets and especially chocolate exacerbate acne. There is really no convincing evidence of this, although if a patient says that they do have an effect it is wise to avoid them. It is therefore not worth imposing a strict diet as this has no proven benefit. However, many pamphlets on acne still advise avoidance of fatty foods, sweets and chocolate.

Before any medical treatment, is there any general advice you could give Shaun?

An optimistic approach is warranted. There is treatment which will improve his acne and so the first thing to do is to point out that today acne is a treatable condition. It is *not* the proper approach to send him away with the retort that he will grow out of it! The adolescent years can be painful enough without the added embarrassment of severe acne. If patients are diligent in the application of therapy (see below), all will be improved and most relieved of the greater part of their acne.

Advice to offer includes:

1. Do not pick the lesions; this spreads the inflammatory material. Do not use comedone extractors because they may damage the skin.
2. Sunlight is of benefit and every opportunity should be taken to enjoy it.
3. Wash at least twice a day with soap and hot water.
4. If girls use cosmetics they should be light and non-greasy, and applied thinly.
5. Try to prevent hair falling over the face. Treat dandruff well.
6. Treatment will take time and persistence.

How would you treat this young man's acne?

Having given the above advice, treatment can be started. Most mild cases of acne respond to topical treatment. I started this boy on a preparation I have found useful, Benoxyl 5 (5% benzoyl peroxide). The benzoyl peroxide preparations (Acetoxyl, Acnegel, Benoxyl, Panoxyl) occasionally give a contact dermatitis; they are keratolytic and antibacterial. I advised him to use it for 2–3 hours only for the first few days to see if any reaction would occur; most patients initially report mild burning with some erythema and scaling of the face in the first 2 weeks, but some seem excessively sensitive and have to be advised to reduce treatment and then gradually increase again. With continued use erythema and scaling seem to disappear. The idea is gradually to increase the treatment to a night-time application to the affected areas, preceded by washing with soap and water. There is also a 10% benzoyl peroxide lotion, but always start with the weaker preparations, saving stronger ones for resistant cases.

An alternative topical preparation is Retin-A gel (tretinoin). As with benzoyl peroxide, start the patient slowly, trying it only for 2–3 hours. With Retin-A gel patients often notice more pustules within 2–3 weeks of use; they must persist. There are new topical retinoids also of use for treating mild to moderate acne, e.g. topical isotretinoin and the retinoid-like adapalene.

Fluorinated steroids are contraindicated, aggravating the condition. Topical antibiotics are increasingly used as alternative treatments for patients with mild acne. Examples are topical erythromycin preparations, (Stiemycin and Zineryt), topical tetracycline solution (Topicycline) and topical clindamycin (Dalacin T). Applied twice daily, they are particularly acceptable to patients in terms of tolerability.

The key to successful treatment with acne lies in persuading the patient to continue the prescribed therapy long enough. It usually responds very slowly and in the first month there may be negligible improvement; but by 3 months there has usually been significant improvement and the patient should continue with the preparation.

Systemic therapy, at the same time as the topical treatment, with a broad-spectrum antibiotic can have very good results—especially in moderately severe acne with papules and pustules. I gave my patient the standard course of oxytetracycline 500 mg b.d. Again it is at least 6 weeks before an effect, and you must continue for 3 months before thinking of changing; erythromycin 500 mg b.d. or minocycline 50 mg b.d. are alternatives if tetracycline fails. Most patients should be kept on the therapy for about 6 months; it must be tailed off slowly. Some doctors put patients on a maintenance dose, e.g. one daily or every alternate day. Certainly further courses or a very long course of treatment may be needed. Remember to advise the patient to take the tetracycline half an hour before meals without milk. Acne can be made worse by strongly progestogenic oral contraceptives and the more oestrogenic pills should be used; with severe acne a change of pill may be considered. Dianette is an agent used for acne which is also a contraceptive but it is wise to reserve this for treating the more moderate/severe forms of acne in young women.

The treatment of acne has been transformed by the introduction of systemic isotretinoin (Roaccutane) therapy. A major teratogen, this treatment is hospital-based and blood tests for liver function and lipids will need to be monitored. Nevertheless, it can be of profound benefit to patients with severe acne.

Are there any conditions which may be confused with acne?

The above is a description of acne vulgaris. There is also an infantile form of acne, and acne can be pro-duced by steroids and certain other drugs. An industrial acne (not a variant of vulgaris) in response to chlorinated hydrocarbons is recognized. There are two principal conditions from which to distinguish acne. The first is perioral dermatitis, and the second is rosacea. Rosacea affects only the face, with erythema, papules and pustules but no comedones. It occurs later in life and diagnosis is not really difficult.

VERRUCAE

A young boy, Terry Glenville, was brought into the surgery one afternoon by his mother. He had a painful foot when he walked because of two small flat circular lesions on the ball of his foot which the mother recognized as verrucae, i.e. plantar warts.

She asked me what causes the warts, whether they would go away without treatment, and if they were contagious, as he was learning to swim? How would you respond?

Warts are caused by viruses. There are different types of wart depending on where they occur. Plantar warts tend to be flat (due to pressure) and circular. Although they do not project they may be very tender. Plantar warts may be single or multiple and they usually have gross hyperkeratosis over the surface. If the lesion is pared down there are characteristic capillary bleeding points distinguishing it from a callosity. A group of warts may combine to form a 'mosaic wart'. Other types of wart include common warts on the hands, which are usually papular, plane warts on the face and neck, anal warts and genital warts.

Warts can disappear without treatment, although it may take months or years; it is impossible to predict. Verrucae are a nuisance and are best treated.

Plantar warts, being viral lesions, are contagious. It has been estimated that 6% of schoolchildren have them. It is usually impossible to stop children passing them on if they are at home, at school or in an institution, but it helps if they cover the wart, use their own towels, bathmats, etc. As for swimming, verrucae are not a reason to avoid learning to swim, provided that they are covered with a waterproof adhesive dressing.

How would you treat Terry's verrucae?

There are numerous ways of treating warts and every doctor has a favourite cure. The one treatment for verrucae that is reasonably clean, effective and well tolerated is treatment with a salicylic acid paint. Formalin, glutarol and other treatments seem less suitable, but every general practitioner supports his or her own remedy and more controlled trials are needed. I prescribed Salactol paint (16.7% lactic acid, 16.7% salicylic acid) for this boy's verrucae, together with corn plasters to ease the pain over the affected areas. I instructed him as follows:

1. Paint the wart then cover with a waterproof plaster and leave 24 hours until the following evening.
2. The following evening take off the plaster, wash and dry the foot and rub vigorously with manicure emery board or pumice stone over the wart.
3. After rubbing apply more paint to the centre of the wart using an orange stick or matchstick (preferable to more conventional applicators). Allow to dry, covering with a further waterproof plaster.
4. Repeat every night without exception.

Printed instructions are helpful. It can take from 6 weeks to 3 months for significant improvement and the patient should be warned that discontinuing the treatment is a major cause of failure. The pain is often soon relieved (especially if corn plasters are used in addition). The wart is healed when the skin appears normal without evidence of a whitish area interrupting the normal skin, however small. If treatment stops before complete cure, recurrence may be a problem. Salactol paint cannot be used on the face; and note that facial warts should not be treated with stronger than 3% salicylic acid paint.

For the treatment of warts in general there are three other alternatives available: (1) curettage, scraping the wart out under anaesthetic, (2) electrocautery and (3) cryocautery. Some general practitioners are now using cryocautery as a quick treatment of verrucae and this should be within the capacity of most large practices.

Table 3.2 lists common varieties of warts and suggests appropriate treatment.

Table 3.2 The treatment of warts

Type of wart	Suggested treatment
Plane facial warts	3% salicylic acid
Multiple periungual warts	Salactol (liquid nitrogen is uncomfortable)
Verrucae (plantar warts)	Salactol or cryocautery
Hand warts	Salactol or cryocautery
Filiform warts on face and neck	Cautery

TEACHING POINTS

1. Acne is a treatable condition.
2. Learn how to prescribe the preparations for acne and what advice to give the patient.
3. Revise the treatment of warts.

THE ELDERLY CONFUSED PATIENT

The care of the elderly is occupying an increasing amount of time in general practice; 18% of consultations in general practice are by patients aged 65 or over. The main problems of the elderly can be summarized as immobility, instability, incontinence and impairment of intellect. Many of the illnesses of the elderly do not present in the classical form, as I found when I was called out to a patient I had last seen 4 years before for a bout of giddiness.

Sarah Woodhouse was an 80-year-old widow. She had been found wandering aimlessly near her home complaining that her house was full of large cats. She had been living on her own for the last 3 years since her husband had died, and a glance at the house revealed that she had considerably neglected herself and her surroundings. There was urine and excrement in the living room and several half-opened tins of food lay on the floor. The carpet was badly frayed. Although it was a warm and sunny day the room was cold. Sarah was very restless and complained of seeing cats everywhere. She knew her name and age, but was disorientated in time and place. There were several old bruises on her arms and legs and a fresh bruise on her occiput. Her clothing was faecally stained and she was incontinent of urine. Examination was difficult. The pulse was 80/min and regular and the BP 130/70, both standing and semirecumbent. She had a carotid bruit on the left. There were no signs of cardiac failure and her chest was clear. The old lady would not stay still long enough for me to palpate the abdomen satisfactorily, although some faecal masses were felt; I thought that trying to perform a rectal examination under these circumstances, although helpful, would have been intrusive and highly disturbing to her. I could not detect any weakness or difference in tone in the arms or legs, but the left plantar response was extensor, the right being flexor. I was unhappy about leaving her at home; I

had not properly made a diagnosis and she had been found wandering in the street. The gas cooker had been left on, and I felt that she was in danger of falling over the scattered furniture. She did not wish to go to hospital, but I decided that she was a real danger to herself and that this warranted compulsory admission. I involved a social worker and a psychogeriatrician and she was admitted to hospital under a Section 2 (see p. 15).

Can a diagnosis be made?

This patient appears to be suffering from a confusional state. She might be suffering from dementia. These two conditions are sometimes difficult to disentangle and, of course, they are not mutually exclusive. The agitation and visual hallucinations point to acute confusion; demented patients tend to be more placid. Another point is that with acute confusion, performance can fluctuate widely and tends to affect all areas of memory and concentration, whereas demented patients often have some memory of their earlier life. Clearly, with the house in such a state all has not been well for a time, so that one may suspect dementia. However, neglect may also be a feature of a depressive illness.

To substantiate a diagnosis of dementia in this patient as well as her current confusion, we need evidence of slow deterioration of intellect over a long period. Neighbours, relatives and friends should be questioned. When dementia is suspected the answers to the following simple questions should be recorded in the notes as they help to establish the level of intellectual function:

- Name?
- Age?
- Date of birth?
- Town?
- Time (to nearest hour)?
- Day?

- Month?
- Year?
- Place at present?
- Address?
- Prime Minister?
- Colour of British flag?

On subsequent visits the scores can be compared. There are also more detailed mental test scores available to document the mental state, e.g. the Mini Mental State Examination and the Abbreviated Mental Test Score.

In this case a neighbour said that for a long time the patient had been vague and forgetful and her appearance had deteriorated over the last 2 years. The likely diagnosis of dementia was in fact later substantiated by the fact that a month after the acute confusion had subsided she was still somewhat disorientated (although less so) and performed poorly in tests of memory, concentration and information. As so often happens, an acute episode has drawn attention to a chronic underlying process.

Dementia must also be distinguished from depression. Once dementia is diagnosed it is important to exclude reversible causes (alcoholism, B12 deficiency, normal pressure hydrocephalus and hypothyroidism). Most cases of dementia are due to Alzheimer's disease (see later).

What causes of an acute confusional state are common?

Confusion in the elderly is a non-specific presentation and a check-list of the more common causes is given in Box 4.1.

This patient had not been on any regular medication (although subsequently several sherry bottles were found in the room). An infection is possible; a urinary tract infection may explain her incontinence. The left extensor plantar may be from an old stroke; in arteriosclerotic or 'multi-infarct' dementia, the dementia may progress by a series of 'little strokes'. Cerebral trauma is a possibility: remember she had bruising on her head. She was not in cardiac failure, but myocardial infarction cannot be ruled out and is often painless in the elderly. There was no arrhythmia, but the presence of a carotid bruit raises the possibility of transient ischaemic attacks (TIAs). Rectal examination may have revealed faecal impaction.

Deafness, blindness and a change of environment all exacerbate confusion and should all be considered. New glasses, a hearing aid and other simple measures may all help.

Could the bruising be significant?

Yes. She had several bruises, including a fresh one on the occiput, and we must remember subdural haematoma as a cause of confusion. This also raises the question, why is she falling? The causes of falls in the elderly make up another useful check-list (Box 4.2). In addition to these the elderly commonly have poor vision (e.g. due to cataract) and dimly lit homes, and chronic confusion often contributes. Dangerous carpets and stairs may cause them to trip.

A patient having TIAs would be considered for aspirin daily, but drug compliance would be poor. Postural hypotension should always be sought as it

---

Box 4.1 Some causes of acute confusion in the elderly

- Drugs (including alcohol)
- Infections
- Cerebrovascular accidents
- Cerebral trauma or tumour
- Hypoxia (including severe anaemia)
- Congestive cardiac failure
- Metabolic causes including uraemia, electrolyte depletion, diabetes mellitus, thyroid disorders
- Constipation (often quoted as a cause)
- Myocardial infarction

Box 4.2 Some causes of recurrent falls in the elderly

- Drop attacks
- Fits
- Transient ischaemic attacks (TIAs)
- Weakness of legs (especially remember CVA, muscle wasting)
- Gait disorders (especially consider Parkinson's disease)
- Postural hypotension (often drug-induced)
- Cardiac disorders, including arrhythmias
- Drugs
- Metabolic causes, including anaemia

is often a remediable cause; advice on getting out of a chair or bed slowly and stopping unnecessary drugs may prove helpful. Cardiac arrhythmias may need to be controlled and there may be a treatable cause for leg weakness, e.g. hypokalaemia, osteomalacia.

Falls always need to be taken seriously in the elderly. They may lead to loss of confidence and hence immobility, with consequent pressure sores, dependent oedema, hypothermia, dehydration or bronchopneumonia. The risk of fracture is always present, with consequent enforced hospitalization.

What is a 'Section 2'?

Section 2 refers to the Mental Health Act 1983 and is one of the forms of compulsory admission to hospital. All general practitioners will need to be acquainted with a few of the more important sections of the Act. As regards compulsory admission to hospital, the two sections below are worth knowing well. Section 4 is to be used where delay would be dangerous.

The reasons for admission on a Section are that the patient is suffering from a mental disorder and ought to be detained in hospital for the interest of his or her own health and safety or with a view to the protection of other people. In this case the gas had been left on and the confusion was such as to prejudice her own safety; you cannot of course apply Section 2 to a person who refuses to go to hospital just because she is uncooperative!

There is a special form to be completed—obtainable from the social worker or psychiatrist. A relative or social worker has to make the application and the other part of the form is completed by the doctor(s). The rules are listed in Table 4.1. Thus a Section 4 (which can be converted to a Section 2 in hospital)

needs only one recommendation, but this must state that it is of urgent necessity that the patient be admitted and application of Section 2 would involve considerable delay.

After a month Mrs Woodhouse was discharged from hospital. The letter indicated that she had had a urinary tract infection, and she had been treated with trimethoprim and an enema for her impaction. She was discharged on lactulose 10 ml nocte and thioridazine for nocturnal restlessness. A diagnosis of acute confusion in a demented patient was made. The hospital had arranged some social support for her. (The general practitioner can equally well arrange this.)

What facilities can the general practitioner arrange for an elderly patient?

General practitioners today work in the context of health care teams. I was able to discuss this patient with the social worker, district nurse and health visitor.

The social worker can advise on financial problems and can also help with many accommodation problems. Financial problems are very important when considering the care of the elderly, and the general practitioner should at least have some idea of the financial help that may be available.

The district nurse performs many duties in the practice; she could help a patient with bathing (and at the same time check that she is taking her medication). Should she need dressings or injections these again would be given by the district nurse. One of the key points of breakdown in any support system is the night-time care. Nocturnal restlessness is particularly difficult for those trying to manage an elderly relative at home, and night nursing facilities are few and far between.

Health visitors will help in assessing a patient's needs and a domiciliary occupational therapy assessment will be useful. The Red Cross can provide many helpful aids in the home.

A very useful facility for the elderly is day care. The aim is to provide some stimulation and company and the centres often provide food and other services (e.g. visits by a chiropodist). A psychogeriatric day unit was used in this case.

A good general practitioner will know the network of support available in the area and the social worker

Table 4.1 Rules for compulsory admission

Application	Medical recommendations	Duration
Section 2 Nearest relative or social worker (approved)	Two (general practitioner and psychiatrist—an 'approved doctor')	Can be detained 28 days for assessment
Section 4 Nearest relative or social worker (approved)	One (preferably a doctor who is acquainted with the patient)	Can be detained 72 hours from admission

Box 4.3 Some services provided by Age Concern, Leicester

1. Advice on social security, rent, rate rebates, improvement grants
2. Information on heating, crime prevention, diets, home safety, savings, investments
3. Furniture removal and refurnishing help
4. Interior decorating
5. Gardening
6. Minor repairs, e.g. to curtain rails
7. Guidance on food supplies and, on special occasions, food parcels
8. Fuel supplies—delivery in an emergency
9. Establishment and support of Drop-In Centres
10. A holiday and leisure bureau

can also be a useful guide to the voluntary agencies, clubs and services available to the elderly. As an example, Box 4.3 outlines some services provided by Age Concern of Leicester. It is important that the general practitioner should regularly review cases such as this in conjunction with other members of the primary health care team.

On reviewing the situation I found that my patient was coping very poorly at home.

What about specific drug treatment?

Anticholinesterases can improve cognition in patients with mild to moderate dementia due to Alzheimer's disease. By delaying the progress of Alzheimer's disease they can help patients stay at home longer. Antipsychotics may be needed to control behaviour/aggression but beware drug side-effects. In particular, try and avoid drugs with anticholinergic side-effects (can worsen Alzheimer's dementia). Newer drugs like risperidone may replace those currently used (promazine, thioridazine, haloperidol). If the patient with dementia is depressed use a selective serotonin reuptake inhibitor (SSRI) not tricyclics.

What are the alternatives?

When elderly people, despite adequate social support, can no longer manage in their own homes, or indeed have nowhere to go, there are a few alternatives open. If they need only a little supervision and can generally look after and feed themselves, then a warden-controlled flat is the answer. If they are not so independent, then a residential home may be the next step to try for.

We are, however, left with the question of what to do for other elderly patients who may be totally immobile, incontinent and/or demented. It is worth noting that 10% aged 65 or over have a significant degree of dementia, 5% severely. Only 1 out of 5 demented patients will be known to their general practitioner. These patients are often a problem and tend to end up as long-stay patients in the hands of the local general hospital or psychiatric hospital. As with residential homes, private nursing homes have expanded in recent years and these, caring as they do for considerably disabled patients, are set to substantially increase the workload of general practitioners in the future. The focus of attention should clearly be with rehabilitation, occupational therapy, active investigation and treatment of difficulties such as falls, incontinence and confusion, in order to keep an elderly person at home as long as possible.

TEACHING POINTS

1. Acute confusion may be due to a treatable cause and is not the same as dementia; distinguish the two.
2. Fully investigate and actively manage confusion, falls and incontinence in the elderly and try to help them maintain independence.
3. Know the procedures for 'Sectioning' a patient.
4. Learn what the facilities are for the elderly in your area.
5. Get to know the other health care professionals attached to your practice and what they have to offer.

5 ABDOMINAL PAIN

Abdominal pain is the fourth most common presenting symptom in general practice and is a considerable challenge to the clinical skills of any doctor. On the one hand, 50% of cases have no identifiable patho-logical cause; on the other hand, 3–4 cases of acute appendicitis may be seen annually by a typical general practitioner. Even in hospital at operation, 30% of cases fail to yield a pathological diagnosis and in those cases there is a correlation with stress and life crises.

A general practitioner's concern is to select those patients who should be referred to hospital for further observation from the 300 or so who will present them-selves in a year and can safely be managed at home or in the surgery.

In the early hours of the morning the phone rang and Mr O'Connor asked whether a doctor would visit his 18-year-old daughter, who had a terrible pain in her stomach.

What questions would you ask?

1. Name, address, age
2. Duration and site of the pain
3. Any vomiting or diarrhoea
4. What is it that worries you most?

These questions will quickly give an outline picture of the problem and allow the doctor to decide whether or not a visit is necessary. Although it is possible in certain circumstances to decline to visit a patient with abdominal pain, such a course of action is fraught with dangers. Unless there are exceptional reasons for such a decision, doctors should visit these patients.

It is important to attempt to assess the degree of urgency of a call like this. Some abdominal cata-strophes can be sudden; requests for visits within half an hour of the onset of pain can place the doctor in a difficult position. It is sometimes wiser to allow a little time to elapse before assessing the pain; colic may abate after half an hour. Not all abdominal pain

Table 5.1 Conditions associated with abdominal pain

Life-threatening conditions which must be excluded	Less urgent but important conditions	Common causes
Appendicitis	Acute cholecystitis	Colic
Acute obstruction	Mesenteric adenitis	Anxiety
Peritonitis	Diabetes	Dietary indiscretion
Ectopic pregnancy	Renal colic	Alcoholic gastritis
Acute pancreatitis	Coronary thrombosis	Gastroenteritis
Twisted ovarian cyst	Acute salpingitis	Migraine
Perforated duodenal ulcer	Acute diverticulitis	Constipation
Strangulated hernia		Dysmenorrhoea
Intussusception (in a child)		Herpes zoster
Sickle cell crisis		
Leaking aortic aneurysm		
Porphyria		

is acute and of recent onset. The presentation may not be as dramatic as in this case.

Common causes of abdominal pain are shown here in Table 5.1. Lists of conditions, if arranged in order of importance, are a useful framework for directing your history and examination.

Mary O'Connor was lying on her side. There was a plastic bowl under the bed.

What questions would you ask?

THE HISTORY

The first step is to take an appropriate history and make a relevant examination. As the examination at this stage rarely reveals much, the history assumes considerable importance.

Stage one   The pain. Questions should be asked about the site, the character, the duration and radiation, factors which relieve, factors which exacerbate, and any other associated symptoms. The patient should be asked what she feels about it.

> **Box 5.1** Check-list of medical conditions which can present as abdominal pain
>
> - Gastric dilatation (diabetic ketosis)
> - Migraine
> - Epilepsy
> - Lead poisoning
> - Tabes dorsalis
> - Addison's disease
> - Haemochromatosis
> - Haemolytic crisis
> - Henoch-Schönlein purpura
> - Hepatoma
> - Hypercalcaemia
> - Uraemia
> - Intestinal parasites

Stage two If the answers to these questions provide any particular clues, further questions should be extended to cover the presence or absence of vaginal discharge, the date of the girl's last menstrual period, and relevant questions about the cardiovascular or respiratory system.

Box 5.1 shows some medical conditions causing abdominal pain.

You obtain a history of low-sided abdominal pain of about 4 hours' duration, not colicky in nature. She has not vomited, and her last period was 2 weeks ago. According to the notes a prescription for oral contraceptives was issued 6 weeks ago.

How do you proceed?

THE EXAMINATION

General examination

1. Signs of pain in her face
2. Her colour
3. The appearance of her tongue
4. The pulse rate
5. The temperature.

Local examination

Examination of the abdomen will be directed towards finding the maximum point of tenderness, the presence or absence of a release sign, whether or not bowel sounds can be heard.

A rectal examination may be indicated if certain conditions are expected, and a vaginal examination,

although rarely indicated, may have to be considered. Such invasive examinations should only be performed when strong indications are found.

At this stage, particularly relevant questions which should have been covered are the presence or absence of haematuria, dysuria and diarrhoea.

Mary was apyrexial, looked pale and anxious and reacted rather violently to the examination. However, the pain was as shown in the Figure 5.1 and not particularly localized. Her abdomen was soft, bowel sounds were present and normal. The release sign was equivocal.

What decision would you now take?

It seems unlikely that Mary has appendicitis but this cannot be excluded. The question of hospital admis-

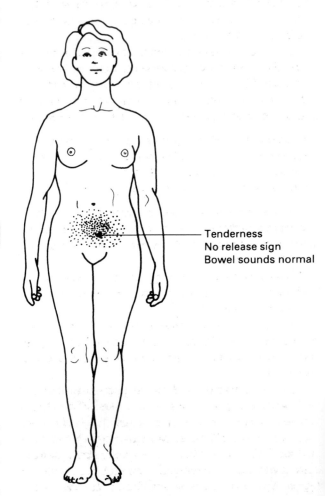

Tenderness
No release sign
Bowel sounds normal

Fig. 5.1 Diagram showing the findings in the accompanying case.

sion must first be considered; in doubtful cases it is not always possible to come to a conclusion at once. Always remember that you can return to see the patient as many times as is necessary in order to make up your mind. On one occasion I remember visiting a boy 4 times before signs of appendicitis became apparent.

If you are in doubt but fairly sure that an abdominal crisis has not occurred it is quite reasonable to return to assess the situation in a few hours. This period of assessment often indicates whether the clinical picture is progressing or subsiding. A further development of symptoms would make the decision to admit to hospital much more likely. On the other hand if they had subsided, further observation will be required.

Clearly the responsibility entailed by observing this case at home is greater than that of referring to hospital, and each individual doctor must have a working hypothesis about the likely cause of symptoms before proceeding. All doctors when genuinely in doubt will refer as a matter of caution.

It is important that the patient herself and her family are taken into consideration when decisions are being made and it is prudent to ask what they fear may be the cause of her problems. A sympathetic approach and an honest appraisal of the situation is needed.

I reassured her that, so far, there were no signs that made me concerned and that careful observation would be the wisest course. I said I would return later in the morning, before surgery.

It is wise to give some indication to the family under what circumstances they are to contact you again. This approach will usually obtain the willing cooperation of all concerned.

Now revise your knowledge of the clinical features of some of the important causes of abdominal pain by studying Table 5.2.

We have now taken the decision to observe the patient at home. If her symptoms become worse it may well be necessary to change our plans and refer her to hospital.

As has been mentioned, the successful management of abdominal pain is based on a view of the likely causes, a high level of suspicion, and early referral for conditions which appear to require hospital investigation. This is coupled with expectant management and reassurance. Appropriate medication should be given for those conditions which are so very much more common and can be safely cared for in the home.

Table 5.2 Cardinal features of major causes of abdominal pain

Cause	Features
Colic	Comes from viscera—exaggerated peristalsis, fades and recurs in cycles
Renal colic	Severity Site—loin Radiation—loin to groin Associated features: vomiting, frequency and dysuria, haematuria
Biliary colic	Site Tenderness maximum in right hypochondrium
Appendicitis	Tenderness History of pain Guarding Temperature raised Vomiting Rectal tenderness
Diverticulitis	Pain Site Tenderness over colon
Peritonitis	Associated with peptic ulceration, acute appendicitis
Peptic ulcer	History Drugs Site of pain Relation to meals Sudden onset Vomiting
Pancreatitis	History Severity Radiation Shock Less rigidity Serum amylase raised

Patients who have normal appendices at operation are found to be twice as likely as controls to have suffered from a severe life crisis in the previous 38 weeks. A gentle enquiry into problems during the last year may offer clues to this situation. Every year in this country some 80 000 operations are performed for appendicitis and some 40 000 of these are found to have histologically normal appendices. If this is the present state of diagnostic certainty in a hospital with full equipment and staff, how much more difficult is the diagnosis at home or in the surgery at a much earlier stage.

In Mary O'Connor's case there is a strong suspicion

that she might be suffering from mild salpingitis because she has recently started on the pill and presumably is now sexually active. There is correlation between abdominal pain, oral contraceptives and sexual activity, and this may be confirmed on examination of the abdomen, by tenderness over the fallopian tubes. A vaginal examination at this early stage will be difficult in the setting of the patient's home, where her early use of contraceptives might not be approved of. A further examination in the surgery could confirm the diagnosis. Swabs should be taken to determine the cause: if not possible refer.

A course of doxycycline and metronidazole would be appropriate if pelvic inflammatory disease is diagnosed.

Later in the morning Mary was sitting up in bed and entirely pain free. It appears that earlier the previous day she had an argument with her boy friend and her father had expressed strong views as to his suitability. I asked her to make an appointment to see me the following day when I could offer her the opportunity to discuss further some of her problems. After her next appointment an MSU grew Escherichia coli sensitive to trimethoprim. I prescribed a 3-day course.

What advice would you give her about her contraceptive?

Rarely, antibiotics alter the action of the pill and ovulation occurs; alternative methods of contraception should be used (see Ch. 11).

TEACHING POINTS

1. Abdominal pain is a challenge and a fine test of clinical maturity.
2. A careful history followed by appropriate examination go far to clarify the situation.
3. A thorough knowledge of the presentation of life-threatening conditions and appropriate check-lists ensure that serious presenting conditions will not be overlooked.
4. Each doctor will have his or her own policy for referral depending on the level of suspicion and knowledge of the patient.
5. It is important to follow up cases of abdominal pain to confirm your diagnosis and to increase your familiarity with the many variations which can occur.
6. Know how to admit a patient to hospital and to make necessary arrangements for transport.

6 CYSTITIS

Cystitis, by which we mean frequency and dysuria, is another of the most common problems presented to a general practitioner. In a practice of 2500 patients, in the region of 60 patients will consult their doctor each year with symptoms suggestive of urinary tract infection. Others have estimated that the symptoms may be responsible for up to 60 per 1000 consultations in general practice and, since it has been shown that only 10% of women with symptoms go to their doctor, cystitis ranks as one of the most common of all human ailments. The majority of patients will be adult women, often with recurrent attacks which may severely curtail their daily activities. It can, however, occur in both sexes and at all ages.

Mrs Baker was a patient well known to the practice, having presented with various problems, of which depression was the most prominent on her recent records. I knew Mrs Baker particularly well; an obese lady, she had been a psychiatric in-patient for 3 years and lived on a small council estate near the surgery. A divorcee with three children, she looked considerably older than her 32 years. She came to the surgery one Monday morning and, after sitting down, requested two lots of tablets—a repeat prescription for her antidepressant and something for her 'cystitis'.

I looked at her notes, dismayed by their thickness. She had, in fact, consulted us twice in the last year for cystitis and on one occasion a mid-stream urine had been sent to the laboratory and had grown Escherichia coli.

Is it worth sending an MSU to document the presence or absence of a urinary tract infection?

In practice, only half the women presenting with dysuria and frequency will have significant bacteriuria ($> 10^5$ organisms/ml of urine) and the terms 'urethral syndrome' and 'frequency and dysuria syndrome' have been used to describe the symptoms of cystitis

---

Box 6.1 Factors precipitating attacks of dysuria and frequency

- Cold weather
- Stress
- The menopause (i.e. oestrogen deficiency)
- Sexual intercourse
- Sensitivity to deodorants and antiseptics (e.g. used in the bath)

---

without a detectable urinary tract infection. There are a variety of factors (Box 6.1) precipitating an attack of frequency and dysuria and these factors alone, in the absence of urinary tract infection, may well explain some cases.

Precipitating factors should be looked for, especially in patients with recurrent symptoms. It is also clear that the criterion of 10^5 organisms/ml is too rigid and a 'negative' report from the laboratory on a mid-stream specimen of urine does not necessarily exclude infection. There are, in addition, a group of patients with symptomless bacteriuria, and the overall prevalence of significant bacteriuria is about 4% in adult women, 0.5% in adult men, 2% in schoolgirls under 12 years old, and less than 1% in preschool children.

Urinary tract infection itself can be regarded as bacteriuria with signs or symptoms. It is usually uncomplicated and confined to the lower urinary tract, the patients presenting with dysuria, frequency, urgency and possibly haematuria. Some patients complain of a suprapubic discomfort. Since recurrent cystitis in adult women, whether associated with proven urinary tract infection or not, has not been shown to lead to deterioration in renal function (raised blood urea, raised blood pressure, renal scarring, etc.), the management of these patients is relatively simple, being largely symptomatic with advice, perhaps a short course of antibiotics and taking particular note of any precipitating factors.

It is doubtful, therefore, that an MSU would contribute significantly to the management of Mrs Baker on this occasion.

Recently, reagent strips for detecting the presence of nitrite, blood and leucocyte esterase in urine have been developed. These can help considerably in deciding on the possibility of a urinary tract infection being present. At least one study has shown that the most accurate method of rapid diagnosis of a urinary tract infection is by low-power microscopy of a drop of urine (Ditchburn R, Ditchburn JS *Br J Gen Pract* 1990; 40: 406–408).

Which antibiotic would be appropriate for Mrs Baker and for how long should the course be prescribed?

Over 80% of uncomplicated urinary tract infections are due to *Esch. coli*. For patients such as Mrs Baker (i.e. non-pregnant adult women with no renal problems) a 3-day course, or even single-dose therapy, has been shown to be just as effective (and cheaper) than the traditional 7- or 10-day course customarily prescribed.

With the increasing resistance of *Esch. coli* to amoxycillin, trimethoprim as a 3-day course or single dose of 400 mg is the treatment of choice. A cephalosporin would be a suitable alternative. Failure to respond to the single or 3-day course would be a reason for requesting an MSU and initiating a longer course of antibiotics. Note that for men, children, pregnant women, those with pyelonephritis, haematuria, diabetes or renal disease, a 7- to 10-day course is still probably advisable.

In sexually active women a chalamydial infection remains a possibility—here a 7- to 14-day course of doxycycline is appropriate. With all patients it is sensible to advise a high fluid uptake and frequent voiding of urine.

Mrs Baker went away with a prescription for trimethoprim but returned 2 months later with a further attack of cystitis—her fourth of the year.

What would be your management now?

As already noted above, there is little evidence of 'recurrent' cystitis causing any lasting damage in the way of deterioration of renal function or elevation of blood pressure. The profitable avenue to explore in the further assessment of Mrs Baker is, therefore, to look at any possible precipitating factors for her cystitis (as outlined in Box 6.1). She is not menopausal so that consideration of oestrogen therapy is inappropriate. I knew that Mrs Baker lived with a man and, since sexual intercourse is a common precipitant, it might be helpful to tactfully offer some advice in this regard (void after intercourse, use lubricants, e.g. KY jelly, to lessen the trauma and, if these fail, try a single dose of nitrofurantoin after intercourse). Mrs Baker should certainly be offered general advice to help alleviate recurrent attacks of cystitis:

1. Avoid deodorants and bath additives.
2. Increase fluid intake and void frequently.
3. Wear stockings rather than tights and cotton rather than nylon underclothes.
4. Discuss contraception—the diaphragm is associated with cystitis, although in this case as far as I was aware Mrs Baker relied on her consort to provide contraception!

Four attacks a year would certainly count as a 'recurrent cystitis' and it would be prudent perhaps to ensure Mrs Baker had some limited form of further assessment in the way of:

1. an MSU—to try to establish if these are now true recurrences of an infection
2. a gynaecological examination
3. a measurement of blood pressure and urea/creatinine on the remote chance of undetected renal problems.

If all these avenues prove to be unhelpful, and Mrs Baker is still troubled by recurring cystitis, it would be worth instituting long-term prophylactic therapy (assuming at least another MSU has documented a true urinary tract infection). Long-term prophylaxis should be continued for at least 6 months. Commonly used prophylactics include nitrofurantoin 100 mg nocte or trimethoprim 100 mg nocte.

Would it be worth referring Mrs Baker for a urological opinion?

It was customary practice to refer women with recurrent attacks of cystitis (i.e. > 3 attacks a year) for a urological opinion but one must adopt a sensible strategy. First one must document that urinary tract infection is indeed the cause—with positive MSUs—and that the 'cystitis' is not a reflection of, say, hormonal deficiency. Second, the patient should have been given an adequate trial of advice and antibiotics. If you are still unable to control the attacks then referral can be considered, and even then it will be more for a urodynamic assessment than an intravenous pyelogram or ultrasonography.

There are, however, groups of patients who do need more active investigation, follow-up and referral. All children with a documented urinary tract infection should be referred—40% of children with a urinary tract infection have an underlying urological tract anomaly of some sort. All males, regardless of age, should be referred for a full assessment (including assessment of the prostate). With women it is advisable to refer for an intravenous pyelogram after an attack of acute pyelonephritis. Urinary tract infection is an important complication of pregnancy and this should be thoroughly documented, treated and followed up during the antenatal course.

TEACHING POINTS

1. Only half the women presenting with dysuria and frequency have significant bacteriuria.
2. A 3-day course, or even single-dose therapy, is effective for uncomplicated urinary tract infections. Trimethoprim is the drug of first choice.
3. All children and all males should be referred after a documented urinary tract infection.
4. Urinary tract infection in pregnancy should be thoroughly documented, treated and followed up during the antenatal course.

7 JOINTS

Sprains and strains take up a good deal of time in practice. Every doctor should be familiar with the examination of the major joints, and in particular in general practice with the shoulder, knee and ankle. Sprained ankles are frequent and shoulder problems may give rise to repeated consultations as progress can be slow. A tennis elbow is not so frequently encountered and even less frequently is it related to tennis! The general practitioner will find a few simple injection techniques useful in dealing with a wide range of joint and local musculotendinous conditions.

SPRAINED ANKLE

A young man, Kevin Gray, came hobbling into the surgery after a bout in the gymnasium saying that he had sprained his ankle. He remembered 'going over' on his ankle and it was now tender and swollen.

What types of ankle sprain are there and is classifying them of any importance?

The sprained ankle requires more thought than it is often given. A simple sprain is a tearing of some fibres of the lateral ligament by an inversion of the foot. The accident usually occurs while walking or running, the foot suddenly inverting. The sprain soon resolves. However, there may be a more severe injury—a complete rather than a partial tear of the lateral ligament (Fig. 7.1). Complete tears may present as severe ankle sprains but the treatment is different. Failure to recognize complete tears may result in recurrent subluxation of the ankle joint so that the ankle 'gives way' and referral for operation may be necessary. Although this is the classical textbook teaching, in practice, as always, things are not as clear-cut. A complete tear is, in fact, rare and the more usual differential diagnosis is a fracture.

It may be very difficult in the acute phase to distinguish complete from partial tears. The complete tear is commonly picked up in 2 weeks after the swel-

Partial tear of the lateral ligament

Complete tear of the lateral ligament

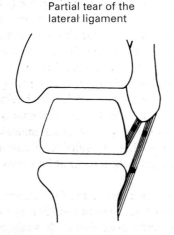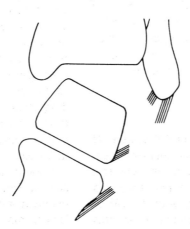

Fig. 7.1 The sprained ankle. Note the excessive movement possible with a complete tear (see text). (Reproduced from Apley (ed.) 1977 *A system of orthopaedics and fractures.* Butterworth, by permission of the publishers.)

ling has resolved or the patient, often a sportsman or sportswoman, presents with an unstable ankle. From the point of view of the general practitioner, therefore, it is more useful to classify ankle sprains as either severe (where there is a possibility of fracture or complete tear) or mild. Four points in the history will help:

1. Swelling. Ask how soon after the injury and how much swelling.
2. Did he carry on with the exercise, sport, etc? If he did, it is unlikely to be severe.
3. Can he now bear weight on the ankle? If he can, it is unlikely to be severe.
4. History of excessive trauma.

What are the signs of a sprained ankle and when would you X-ray the ankle?

The signs of a sprained ankle vary considerably in severity and in many cases there is only a mild tenderness. The signs include:

1. swelling of the ankle, mainly on the lateral side
2. bruising may occur
3. tenderness, maximal around the site of the lateral ligament
4. inversion of the ankle is painful
5. in complete tears there may be excessive movement.

A complete lateral ligament tear occurs with a violent inversion injury—there is rapid swelling and there may be extensive bruising. Both complete and partial lateral ligament tears are tender, but walking is usually impossible with the complete tear. Test the movement of the ankle gently—while both will have pain on inversion, there may be excessive movement with the complete tear. Often, however, severe pain prevents testing a full range of movement. Be sure to palpate all bony prominences to detect a local fracture.

X-rays

It is important to note that both plain AP and lateral radiographs will be normal in lateral ligament tears. To distinguish between a partial and a complete tear, 'strain films' are needed, whereby X-rays are taken with both ankles inverted (possibly with the aid of an anaesthetic); if the ligament is ruptured the talus

will tilt medially. Hence in severe sprains, where there is excessive movement or you are unable to examine due to pain, an X-ray should be considered. Furthermore, an X-ray will exclude a fracture. With a fracture the ankle may be very swollen with a variable site for the tenderness and limited ankle movement.

The indications for X-ray can be summarized thus:

- No X-ray: simple sprains
- X-ray: possible fracture, e.g. tenderness elsewhere
  severe signs (swelling, bruising etc)
  unusual movement of ankle
  unable to examine due to pain
  simple sprains not responding
  history of excessive trauma.

How would you treat this patient?

He had a little swelling over the lateral ligament but minimal tenderness and no bruising. He could walk on his foot and movement was normal; I diagnosed a simple sprain.

The main treatment of simple sprains is to provide good support to the ankle with elastic adhesive strapping (e.g. Elastoplast or Tubigrip); crepe bandages when applied do not provide sufficient support and are inferior. Initially ice will help to ease the pain. The correct way to apply strapping is something that needs to be learnt and the mere prescription of strapping without instructions is like prescribing a drug without advice. Preferably the practitioner should apply the strapping personally or delegate the task to an experienced nurse. I start with a stirrup and then apply the strapping from the inner side of the sole of the foot across the outer side of the foot and then up the ankle and leg as far as the tibial tubercle. There should be a resultant mild eversion of the ankle after strapping. In the first day elevation will help and non-weight-bearing exercises of plantar and dorsiflexion should be started at once. A non-steroidal anti-inflammatory drug should be prescribed (if not contraindicated) to reduce pain and swelling. If available, ultrasound is very valuable. All ankle sprains must be reviewed in 2 weeks.

If the patient does not exercise the joint following an ankle sprain, adhesions may form and this may even require manipulation under anaesthesia. Physiotherapy is very important after an ankle sprain.

A complete tear will be diagnosed in hospital on referral of the severe sprain. It may be treated by immobilization in a padded plaster. If a complete tear has been missed, presents late or is inadequately treated as a simple sprain, the ligament can fail to repair and an operation may be needed, as already noted above.

TENNIS ELBOW

William Wallace, a garage mechanic, complained of pain over the lateral side of his elbow. It had been present, he thought, for about 3 weeks, was not getting any better, and was beginning to interfere with his work which involved a lot of lifting and intricate manoeuvres. After examination I decided that he had a 'tennis elbow'.

What are the normal features of a 'tennis elbow'?

Tennis elbow is the most common of the elbow conditions seen in practice and is found in any occupation in which the forearm is used a lot, for example, housework. The main pathology is damage to the common extensor origin with the resultant adhesions of fibres around the site. It is seen most commonly among young or middle-aged patients and the onset is usually insidious.

The patients' complaints are usually centred on the fact that they cannot do their jobs properly because of pain with certain movements. The diagnosis can often be made by the movement which is most painful, as these movements will be the ones putting the greatest strain on the common extensor origin; thus with a housewife it may be pouring the tea or dusting, with a squash player his backhand may suffer, and the workman may find using a screwdriver difficult.

There are three principal features to note:

1. There is localized tenderness over the lateral epicondyle at the point of the muscle attachments.
2. There is pain on resisted dorsiflexion of the wrist with elbow straight and forearm pronated; this is the most useful clinical test in the surgery.
3. The elbow looks normal and the range of movements is full.

Nothing will be shown on X-ray; it is normal. There is little of importance as a differential diagnosis, but remember that cervical spondylosis can present as an atypical tennis elbow.

What is the available treatment?

The usual course of a tennis elbow is natural recovery, but it can take many months and the prognosis for each tennis elbow is so variable that treatment is warranted.

Injection therapy is most useful and so is physiotherapy; if both fail then referral will probably be necessary.

Rest and injection therapy

Rest is important and rest in a sling will alleviate some of the pain. Injection therapy is well within the scope of the average practitioner. The technique is best learnt from practical experience but there are several tips to improve your success rate. There is a choice of preparations to inject. You can use a mixture of 1% lignocaine (2–3 ml) and 1 ml (25 mg) of hydrocortisone acetate or longer-acting steroids, e.g. methylprednisolone (Depo-Medrone) or triamcinolone acetonide (Kenalog). Atrophic changes in the subcutaneous tissues are an occasional problem with these longer-acting preparations. It is worth warning patients of the possibility of depigmentation following a steroid injection. As regards technique the following advice may be useful:

1. Inject first at the point of greatest tenderness at the origin of the forearm extensor muscles from the lateral epicondyle. All areas of pain around the tendon insertion must be infiltrated at one injection so that slightly altering the angle of the needle will cover other points.
2. Inject under pressure.
3. Inject down to the periosteum of bone.
4. The injection itself should be mildly painful, and reinsert down to bone a few times without withdrawing.
5. Warn the patient that pain may actually be exacerbated for 24 hours after the injection.

Figure 7.2 summarizes the injection technique. The pain should ease in a few days. Ask the patient to come back in 2 weeks if no better, resting the elbow in the meantime. If no better, then try a second injection. With hydrocortisone acetate the effect seems to wear off sooner and we are now changing to the

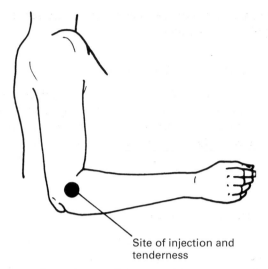

Site of injection and
tenderness

Fig. 7.2 Injecting a tennis elbow. Using a blue or green needle, inject 1% lignocaine and steroid (see text) into the site of maximal tenderness. Inject deep, down to the bone, and under pressure reinsert a few times without withdrawing, infiltrating widely.

use of Depo-Medrone injection because of its longer action.

Physiotherapy

If three injections have failed, I would ask the physiotherapist for help. The physiotherapist can help with massage, short-wave diathermy and ultrasound. There is no reason, of course, why physiotherapy techniques should not be employed at the outset—much depends on access. Some enthusiasts of manipulation claim successes with tennis elbow.

Rest in plaster

Textbooks often mention rest in plaster, but this is not very practical for most people. The effects of keeping an elbow in plaster must be such that it could take a time to recover full range of movement, thus substituting one disability for another.

Surgery

In a few persistent and recurrent cases an operation on the extensor origin is necessary.

The approach to tennis elbow will thus differ slightly from doctor to doctor.

In the case of this mechanic, after two injections he was back working as hard as ever.

PAINFUL SHOULDER

A 50-year-old building foreman, Albert Oakfield, came to the surgery complaining of a painful shoulder. His history was that he had been lifting about 4 weeks previously and thought he had 'sprained' his shoulder at the time. He was used to sprains in his line of work and had thought little of it, but gradually the shoulder had become more painful, especially with some movements, so that his ability to lift and carry had been severely limited. His firm was very busy and he said he had to work on and could not afford to rest. 'Is there anything you can do to help the pain?' he asked.

What are the main causes of shoulder pain? Outline briefly a quick examination of the shoulder joint which you would carry out in the surgery.

For revision, the main causes of a painful shoulder are outlined in Table 7.1.

It does not take long to examine a shoulder in practice, but as a reminder the following is a typical guide.

A. Inspection

Look at the bony contours and alignment. Is there any swelling?
In long-standing conditions, is there any muscle wasting?

B. Palpation

Feel bony and soft tissue parts for any areas of tenderness.

C. Movements

1. Ask the patient to raise both arms sideways with palms facing upwards until they point directly upwards and then lower them again (*abduction*).
2. Ask the patient to touch the opposite shoulder blade by moving the arm in front of the body (*adduction*) and then behind the back (*internal rotation*).

Table 7.1   Causes of a painful shoulder

Condition		Notes
1. Arthritis:	pyogenic	Uncommon
	osteoarthritis	Uncommon; can get OA of acromioclavicular joint giving painful abduction
	rheumatoid	Look for other evidence of RA
	tuberculous	Rare
2. Musculotendinous cuff lesions (including 'painful arc' syndrome)		Common. A 'mixed bag' of pathology; largely tears and tendinitis of the supraspinatus tendon and subacromial bursitis
3. Trauma:	sprains fractures dislocation	
4. Bicipital tendinitis		Tendinitis in the bicipital groove
5. Referred pain:	a. from the neck	Cervical disc lesions and cervical spondylosis, relatively common. Pain and restriction on neck movement
	b. other	Myocardial ischaemia, neoplasm of bronchus, diaphragmatic irritation
6. Herpes zoster		During prodromal phase when affecting cervical root ganglia
7. Polymyalgia rheumatica		In elderly, typically morning stiffness and aching in neck, shoulders, arms. Constitutional upset, ESR raised
8. Frozen shoulder		May follow cuff lesions. All movements restricted. Goes through three phases—increasing pain and stiffness, then stiff but little pain, and finally return of movement with no pain (provided shoulder has not been immobilized). Whole course may last up to 2 years
9. Shoulder—hand syndrome		Shoulder painful and stiff. Same hand also affected and may be swollen with shiny atrophic skin. Obscure aetiology; may follow myocardial infarction

3. Ask the patient to flex his elbows with them firmly pressed into his sides and then to separate the hands (*external rotation*).

4. Raising the arm forwards and backwards tests *flexion* and *extension*. In (1)–(4) note diminution of range of movement and note pain when it occurs.

5. Passively move the shoulder through its range of movement.

6. The movements can be tested against resistance—in particular test abduction, external rotation and internal rotation.

7. If bicipital tendinitis is suspected, resisted flexion of the forearm should be tested.

8. Remember in assessing movement of the shoulder joint that a lot of movement can be attributed to scapula movement. It is important to eliminate this rotation of the scapula, especially in abduction, as even when the shoulder joint is relatively 'frozen' some movement in abduction will be caused by scapula rotation.

9. When there is a full range of movement and/or any suggestion of pain radiating from the neck, test movements of the cervical spine (flexion, extension, rotation, lateral flexion); testing the cervical spine completes the examination proper of a painful shoulder.

The above examination will usually permit diagnosis by the pattern of restriction of movement and pain. In a frozen shoulder all movements may be limited. Occasionally when the pain is real and local examination negative, more general examination will be needed.

On examination of Mr Oakfield the most consistent finding was of pain experienced on abduction, but only after the first 60° or so until about 120°, i.e. there was a painful arc. There was also a point of deep tenderness around and below the acromion process.

What are the causes of the 'painful arc' syndrome? Describe it more fully.

The 'painful arc' syndrome is a fairly specific disorder. With the arm at the patient's side there is little, if any, pain but on abduction of the arm to about 60° pain is felt and persists until about 120° is reached, at which point the pain disappears. When the arm is brought down pain is felt again over this mid-abduction range (Fig. 7.3).

The 'painful arc syndrome' is said to be caused by a variety of minor lesions, including (1) incomplete tear of the supraspinatus tendon, (2) supraspinatus tendinitis, (3) calcification of the supraspinatus tendon, (4) subacromial bursitis, (5) fracture of the greater tuberosity. Osteoarthrosis of the acromioclavicular joint is said to give superficially similar symptoms. In reality most could well be small tears of the supraspinatus tendon. The supraspinatus lesions are part of the musculotendinous or rotator cuff lesions which are quite common causes of a painful shoulder in family practice. It is very doubtful if the average practitioner can or indeed needs to distinguish between the above lesions.

be necessary if pain is still severely incapacitating the patient.

List some common sites where injections may be of use

These are shown in Table 7.2. All the conditions listed should be well within the competence of the average practitioner to treat. All in the list are common and the reader would find it profitable to look up the conditions and learn the relevant techniques as appropriate. It may be found helpful to make a little card of each condition and keep them by the trolley used for injections; on each card can be put (1) treatment options, (2) if injection indicated, where and what to inject, (3) follow-up required.

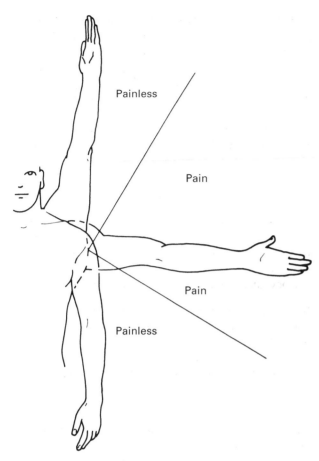

Fig. 7.3 The painful arc syndrome; diagram to demonstrate pain occurring in the mid-abduction range.

Table 7.2 Some common sites where injections may be of use

Site	Condition
Shoulder	Supraspinatus tendinitis
	Subacromial bursitis
	Frozen shoulder
	Bicipital tendinitis
Elbow	Tennis elbow
	Golfer's elbow
Wrist and hand	Carpal tunnel syndrome
	De Quervain's tenosynovitis
	Trigger finger
Knee	Prepatellar bursitis
Foot	Plantar fasciitis

How would you manage this patient?

There are three things that will help: (1) heat, e.g. short-wave diathermy, (2) exercise—using the arm as much as possible, (3) injection therapy.

Using aseptic technique, I used a large needle to inject the shoulder via the lateral approach, feeling for the lateral tip of the acromion and inserting the needle below the acromion process in a medial direction. Again the choice is 1% lignocaine plus hydrocortisone or Depo-Medrone. After penetrating 2.5–5 cm (1–2 inches) you can infiltrate, after first aspirating to exclude pus, and it may reproduce the symptoms; if it does not, altering the angle of the needle slightly may help. Using the above technique, after a few minutes the pain may be much relieved. The injection can be repeated in 3 weeks. If this fails, an operation may

TEACHING POINTS

1. Distinguish between severe and mild ankle sprains.
2. X-ray severely sprained ankles.
3. Treatment depends on severity of the sprain, but for simple minor sprains it consists of elastic adhesive strapping and early exercise.
4. Tennis elbow is a common elbow condition occurring with people from many occupations.
5. Learn how to inject a tennis elbow.
6. Revise the causes of a painful shoulder and practise a quick efficient method for examining the shoulder joint in your surgery.
7. Learn injection techniques for other musculotendinous conditions encountered in general practice.

8 THE PAINFUL EAR

About one quarter of all children will see their general practitioner at some time with earache or impaired hearing. Consulting rates for acute otitis media are 120 per year for a list of 2000 patients or 600 per year for a list of 10 000 patients. Otitis media with effusion is the most common cause of hearing loss; it occurs in 20% of children around the age of 2 years, with another peak at the age of 5.

Otitis media usually starts with an upper respiratory infection leading to inflammation which blocks the eustachian tube. Fluid collects in the middle ear, which then becomes infected with bacteria or viruses from the nose. Within hours the patient develops earache followed, if it worsens, by severe pain, malaise and fever. There can be a discharge from the ear and/or giddiness. Eighty per cent of cases resolve without treatment within about 3 days; the symptoms subside and the ear drum remains intact. If, however, the pressure of the effusion rises, the pain will get worse and the drum perforates, allowing the fluid to run into the external meatus. When this occurs the pain suddenly disappears, although deafness will persist until the drum heals again.

Mrs Chilterman brought her 4-year-old son, Mark, to the surgery one morning saying that he had been crying all night and holding his ear.

What questions would you ask?

- Where is the pain? Is it in the ear, behind the ear, or below the ear? Is it one ear or both ears? Is it a severe pain or a mild pain? How long has it been there?
- Have there been any other features, such as sore throat, vomiting or diarrhoea, temperature, runny nose or a discharge from the ear?
- Has he been noticed to be deaf? Is he vomiting, complaining of a headache or giddiness?
- Has he ever had anything like this before?

- Is he a contact of anyone with either a respiratory tract infection or any other infectious disease?
- A prudent question at this stage would be to find out whether he is allergic to penicillin.

The answers to all these questions are unhelpful. He merely has a pain in his ear and seems a little hot.

What examination would you make?

Examination of the ear is a skill that is acquired by practice, and a registrar should take every opportunity to perfect the ability to examine the ears of children from the very earliest age upwards. It is usually possible to perform this without causing undue stress

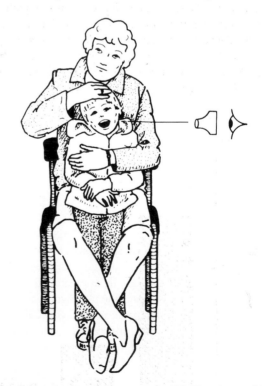

Fig. 8.1 Position in which a parent should hold a reluctant child or infant for the examination of the ears, nose or throat.

(Fig. 8.1). The main object of the examination is to try to visualize the drum. Additional examination may consist of noting whether there is tenderness on traction of the pinna, the presence or absence of a discharge and whether there is any tenderness over the mastoid process. Be careful not to inflict pain with the end of the auriscope.

On examination you find that Mark has an entirely red drum with loss of light reflex but no obvious bulging.

How would you now manage him?

RAPRIO is a useful acronym when thinking of various aspects of management and it will be used here as an illustration.

R *Reassure* Mrs Chilterman that you have found an infection in her sons's ears and that adequate treatment with an antibiotic will cure it. Explain this to Mark also.
A *Advise* the mother to give him plenty of fluids, especially if he is pyrexial, and to use Calpol if he is in pain. It is also important to stress that the medicine should be given until the course is completed.
P *Prescribe* amoxycillin 125 mg t.d.s. for a week after checking that there is no history of allergy. I make a point of giving the prescription to the child and saying, 'I want you to take this medicine until it is all gone.'

R *Referral* is not necessary unless there is tenderness over the mastoid process and the ear is protruding.
I *Investigations* (e.g. a swab if discharge present) are unlikely to help your management at this stage.
O *Observe*. See the patient in a week to check that the inflammation is subsiding. Ask the mother to bring him back after about 4 weeks if she thinks that he might be deaf.

Long-term complications are:

1. glue ear (otitis media with effusion)
2. deafness
3. chronic suppurative otitis media.

Other complications of otitis media include acute mastoiditis and meningitis. Rarely persistent infection can cause intracranial sepsis or facial palsy.

ACUTE OTITIS MEDIA

By far the most common cause of a painful ear in children is otitis media. The presentations are shown in Figure 8.2.

This is an inflammation of the middle ear cleft. There is a familial factor and the incidence is inversely related to the social class of the patient. Pain is a very common accompanying feature and infants may present with nothing except malaise, vomiting or screaming

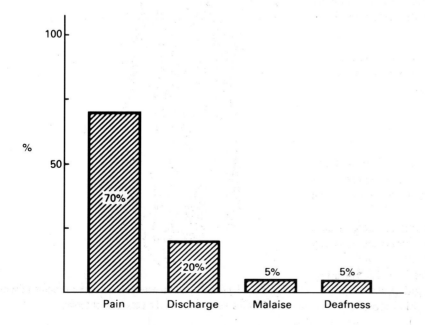

Fig. 8.2 Proportional representation of presenting symptoms of otitis media.

attacks. The condition is secondary to an upper respiratory tract infection and more common in the winter months. The diagnostic feature is the appearance of a red drum. The inflammatory process usually begins in the upper posterior quadrant and spreads peripherally and down the handle of the malleus (see Fig. 8.3).

The appearance of a bulging drum is a late feature. Blisters may often be seen on the tympanic membrane and this is thought to be due to a virus infection in the epidermal layers of the drum.

The differential diagnosis is from other causes of pain in the ear such as foreign bodies, tonsillitis, dental problems and occasional temporomandibular arthritis in an older age group. The most common infecting organisms encountered in the upper respiratory tracts of children are illustrated in Figure 8.4.

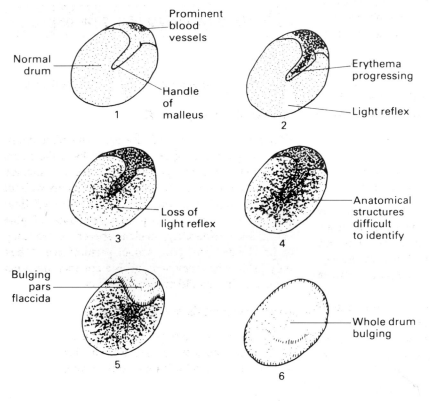

Fig. 8.3 Stages in the progress of an acute otitis media of the right tympanic membrane.

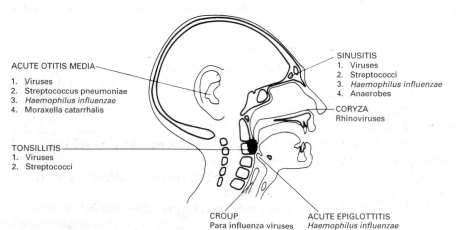

ACUTE OTITIS MEDIA
1. Viruses
2. Streptococcus pneumoniae
3. *Haemophilus influenzae*
4. Moraxella catarrhalis

TONSILLITIS
1. Viruses
2. Streptococci

CROUP
Para influenza viruses

ACUTE EPIGLOTTITIS
Haemophilus influenzae

SINUSITIS
1. Viruses
2. Streptococci
3. *Haemophilus influenzae*
4. Anaerobes

CORYZA
Rhinoviruses

Fig. 8.4 Infections of the upper respiratory tract; sites and common organisms.

The treatment of choice for patients with otitis media is amoxycillin, as this is more active than penicillin against *Haemophilus influenzae*. With increasing resistance and β-lactamase production by some bacteria, co-amoxiclav is now favoured by some. If the patient is allergic to penicillin, erythromycin can be used. A classic study by Jones & Bain (*J R Coll Gen Pract* 1986; 36:356) has shown that a 3-day course of antibiotics is sufficient. Some argue that, since many cases of otitis media are viral in origin, mild cases can be managed with analgesia alone. In the Netherlands, for example, most children with acute otitis media are managed without antibiotics.

Antibiotics are recommended for younger children (e.g. under age 3), children who are systemically ill or who have a perforated drum with a discharge. Children with recurrent attacks should also be treated with antibiotics.

What are the problems presented to the general practitioner by an attack of acute otitis media?

Difficulty in making a diagnosis. This is unusual except in babies. There is rarely difficulty in establishing the diagnosis once the drum is inspected, but the presence of wax can be a hindrance. Allergy to penicillin may force a choice to be made between other suitable antibiotics.

The danger of spread of infection to the mastoid bone is now fortunately very rare. Cases of meningitis associated with otitis media must be borne in mind, especially in the very young and those with immunological impairment.

Persistent deafness is perhaps the most difficult complication to manage and the role of antibiotics in the aetiology of (otitis media with effusion) glue ear is still debatable.

The purpose of any follow-up must be to detect those ears which have not resolved within a reasonable period of time. The majority will have no detectable deafness after 3 weeks. In one study in general practice there was no difference between children who were thought to be deaf by their parents, those who were thought to be deaf by their general practitioner and those who were found to be deaf by routine audiometric screening. Thus it is reasonable to follow up only those who are perceived to have deafness and to ask parents to bring back any child in whom they noticed deafness after 4 weeks.

The commonly held view, however, is that one should review the drum and hearing after 3 weeks.

The roles of the School Health Service and health visitor in routine screening for deafness may be regarded as complementary and aim to detect those with approximately a 15 decibel loss as demonstrated by audiometry. This detects those with otitis media with effusion and other forms of deafness who have not been identified by other means.

GLUE EAR (OTITIS MEDIA WITH EFFUSION)

Definition

A chronic accumulation of fluid in the middle ear.

What should our response be?

Children who present with deafness, and other symptoms suggestive of glue ear, should have their ears examined. Specific symptoms of glue ear include earache (but more commonly deafness occurs without earache), tugging at the ears and a sense of fluid moving in the ear. Non-specific symptoms of glue ear include irritability, unclear speech, a tendency to be isolated and poor school performance. 'They only listen when they want to' is a common maternal comment that should arouse suspicion.

Signs to be seen with the auriscope

- Cloudy/milky drum, perhaps retracted
- Fluid may be seen as a level or bubbles
- There is often a bluish hue to the drum.

Treatment
A prolonged (4–8 weeks) course of antibiotics may aid resolution.

When to refer
If there is no resolution after 3 months refer for insertion of grommets to allow drainage of the fluid.

TEACHING POINTS
1. The ability to examine the ear of a child is a skill which should be acquired.
2. Appropriate antibiotic treatment for sufficient time reduces complications.
3. Follow up those children who appear to be deaf.

9 CHEST PAIN

Chest pain can be one of the most challenging and difficult presentations with which a doctor is faced. It epitomizes the aphorism that common things occur commonly. There is an increasing awareness amongst the general population of the possible significance of chest pain, and epidemiologically there is ample evidence of rapidly increasing death rates in coronary artery disease. What information is needed to give a sense of proportion against which to weigh the probabilities?

Five per cent of the population had pain in the chest within a 2-week study period. There was no difference between men and women and it occurred at all ages. A general practitioner may expect 2–3% of new patients to complain of pain in the chest. In less than half these cases has a diagnosis been made by the doctor.

In the average general practice this means 94 consultations a year, or two new presentations a week. Of the 5% who have chest pain in the population, half consult their doctor. Cardiovascular disease accounts for 51% of all deaths in Great Britain and the United States. Nearly 300 000 patients will have a myocardial infarction in the UK every year.

In a practice of 2500 patients, the picture might be as in Table 9.1.

Coronary heart disease represents 17% of all cardiovascular disease. An average general practitioner may expect 14% of all patients who consult to have cardiovascular disease. This represents 8% of the population

at risk. Myocardial infarcts represent 5 per 1000 population at risk in a year, and the male to female ratio is 2.5 to 1.0.

CENTRAL CHEST PAIN IN ISCHAEMIC HEART DISEASE

The World Health Organization definition of cardiac pain is as follows:

> In the front of the chest, mid or upper sternum radiating to the left arm or both arms, round the chest or into the jaw. Rarely of more than 30 minutes duration unless a coronary thrombosis has occurred. The words used to describe it are: tight, heavy, constricting, crushing, numbing or burning.

When the cause is in doubt the examination is rarely helpful and the history is of most value. Patients have difficulty in describing what they feel; they need time. Non-verbal clues, the movements of the hand, the clenching of their fists, should be closely observed. Their past history and previous behaviour will be very helpful. The statistics of this incidence of ischaemic heart disease, given in Table 9.1, should help in forming judgements about individual patients.

An ex-miner, George Whittington, in his early 60s, has chest pain. He last consulted you 7 years ago when he had a diaphragmatic hernia repaired. His present trouble is that he has noticed a retrosternal pain for 3 days. It is not related to anything, but he has heaviness in his arms. He is a smoker and he is well cared for by his wife.

How should you assess this chest pain?

The important points in the history are the site of the pain, its quality and intensity, the time sequence

Table 9.1 Cardiovascular disease seen in a practice of 2500 patients in a year

Disease	Number seen
Raised blood pressure	50 (one a week)
Angina	11 (one a month)
Myocardial infarct	8 (one in 6 weeks)
Other ischaemic heart disease	13 (one a month)
Total	82

and duration, and the factors affecting it, e.g. eating, exercise, breathing or movement. Secondary features such as sweating, vomiting, other symptoms, and his approach to his condition are also important. A past history of similar events and a drug history, whether he is working, and his smoking habits, are all most relevant.

Today the pain has been present continuously for several hours; it is like a tight band across the whole of his chest and he feels something in his throat. He has tried proprietary analgesics to no avail. He has had similar pains in the past few weeks when he walked back to his house from the pub, but these disappeared when he rested.

What examination should you now make?

Some clothing should be removed in order to facilitate a proper assessment. He has an indoor pallor. He is not anaemic and is sweating. His pulse is 110; his blood pressure 180/115; he is slightly dyspnoeic and there are no signs in his chest; he has no ankle oedema and his jugular venous pulse is not raised. Heart sounds are normal.

What diagnoses will you consider?

It is important to remember that any structure in the chest can give rise to pain. Table 9.2 shows important causes of chest pain other than ischaemic heart disease and their distinguishing features.

How would you proceed?

The nature of the pain and its distribution and duration are suggestive of a recent myocardial infarct. His previous history of a repaired hiatus hernia suggests the possibility of reflux oesophagitis, but the nature of the pain and the fact that it is not affected by food and that he has no history of indigestion are points against this. You make a presumptive diagnosis of myocardial infarct. The decision now most pressing is whether he should be managed at home or in hospital. In recent years, with the arrival of thrombolytic therapy and new antiarrhythmic protocols, the balance has swung towards hospital care for all patients with a myocardial infarction. General practitioners clearly may have to temper this view with some consideration for the extremes of age and infirmity, but as a rule

Table 9.2 Causes of chest pain

Cause	Features
Pericarditis	May mimic myocardial infarction, worse on inspiration. Tamponade with paradoxical pulse and raised jugular venous pressure rare. A friction rub which may be scratchy. ECG changes—concave ST elevation. Needs investigation
Aneurysm	Tearing sensation radiating to the back, hemiparesis, loss of pulse, shock. Possible cause—Marfan's syndrome. X-ray shows characteristic changes
Pulmonary embolus	Sudden chest pain, central, hypotension, dyspnoea, cyanosis, right heart strain, ECG, pleuritic pain, haemoptysis. Chest X-ray can be unhelpful. Often associated with deep vein thrombosis, varicose veins and/or contraceptives
Spontaneous pneumothorax	Pain and dyspnoea. At any age. Think of this especially in young people. Mediastinal shift and tension. Hyperresonance. Chest X-ray essential
Oesophageal pain	Reflux with hiatus hernia. May mimic cardiac pain. Heartburn easy to distinguish. Burning, acid pain, after meals, especially on bending. Relieved by alkalis
Spinal pain	Degenerative changes, root pain, related to movement specifically. X-ray is helpful but after the age of 50 many have some changes

patients should be admitted. Mr Whittington, a still sprightly 64-year-old, was referred to hospital. There is still, however, a lot a general practitioner can do with a patient having an acute myocardial infarction while awaiting transportation to the hospital (Box 9.1).

Mr Whittington had had a small myocardial infarction and was discharged from hospital 1 week later on aspirin and a beta-blocker. How would you advise him?

Mr Whittington smoked 10 cigarettes per day and clearly this is the major area for discussion—smoking must cease. All patients' postmyocardial infarction should be considered for four drugs:

1. A beta-blocker—this reduces the risk of death and reinfarction by 25% (providing no contraindications).
2. Aspirin (150–300 mg/day)—this also reduces the risk of death and reinfarction (providing there are no contraindications).
3. An ACE inhibitor if heart failure is present.
4. A statin. Post myocardial infarction the LDL cholesterol should be reduced to <3.2 mmol/l

Box 9.1 The general practice management of a patient with a myocardial infarct

1. Use of defibrillators. Ventricular fibrillation is the usual cause of death in patients with a myocardial infarction and its early recognition and treatment can save lives. General practitioners should consider carrying a portable defibrillator, especially in rural areas

2. Analgesia. The analgesia of choice is diamorphine 5 mg intravenously, with 2.5 mg i.v. given at 10 minute intervals. Prochlorperazine (Stemetil) should be given as an antiemetic (by injection)

3. Aspirin. Unless sensitive to aspirin, or there is a known contraindication, all patients should be given 150 mg of aspirin—this simple measure will reduce mortality by 25%

4. Nitrolingual spray. Use of a nitrate spray will help a patient with an acute myocardial infarction

5. Treatment of:
   a. arrhythmias e.g. bradycardia (50–60 beats/min) with 0.3–0.6 mg i.v. of atopine
   b. left ventricular failure with i.v. frusemide.

6. Thrombolytic therapy. It has been conclusively demonstrated that i.v. thrombolytic therapy, e.g. with antistreplase (Eminase), can significantly reduce mortality from myocardial infarction if given in the early stages (within the first 6 hours). Providing there is no tendency to bleed (including conditions such as a peptic ulcer where haemorrhage is a risk), there are powerful arguments for general practitioners to administer these thrombolytics in the acute stage

(total serum cholesterol to <4.8 mmol/l). At about 3 months post infarction, Mr Whittington should have his cholesterol measured.

Mr Whittington has been prescribed a beta-blocker and aspirin and these should continue. He should be advised to follow a sensible diet and he should be advised against driving for 2 months. A cardiac rehabilitation programme (with a series of graduated exercises, some counselling and self-help groups) is valuable if locally available.

When considering chest pain remember:

1. Twenty per cent of patients with coronary thrombosis complain of previous angina.

2. A patient with new angina getting worse has a 1 in 6 chance of developing coronary thrombosis.

TEACHING POINTS

1. Chest pain is a great challenge:
   (a) Any structure in the chest can produce pain.
   (b) Coronary thrombosis is a major disease of our time.
2. Diagnosing a coronary is not nearly as clear-cut as it may seem with hindsight and we are frequently surprised.
3. Many patients are fully aware of the significance of chest pain and are not always reassured by our examination of them.
4. Careful history and examination are the cornerstones of management.
5. The exclusion of a coronary is a large part of our task.
6. Coronary thrombosis should not blind us to other causes.
7. Appropriate investigations can be very useful both as an exclusion and in making a diagnosis.
8. Too ready assurance is counterproductive.
9. Become conversant with the new medical management of patients with a myocardial infarction.

10 HEART FAILURE

Based on a commissioned article for *Horizons* 28 July 1989 (reproduced with permission) and updated in 1998.

How often does it occur?

Heart failure is relatively uncommon. A general practitioner with 2000 patients can expect to have in his or her care 22 persons with this condition in a year. Of these, 12 will have congestive heart failure, two left ventricular failure, two cor pulmonale and six cardiac arrythmias. Each will generate five or six consultations. The annual consulting rate rises dramatically with age from 5 or 6 per 100 cases at 45 years to 75 per 100 cases at 75 years of age.

Mr Greenwood, a new patient, presented himself at my surgery one morning. He had returned from holiday early because he was short of breath. He asked to be seen on the ground floor as he could not face the stairs. He was sitting down as I entered and I saw a man in his late 50s with a plethoric complexion and a slight bluish tinge. He was sitting in a somewhat 'Churchillian' posture, panting for breath.

What questions would you ask?

In this article only the questions relevant to a heart condition are considered. Mine were:

- History of present complaint?
- How long have you been like this?
- Have you had this before?
- Have you noticed any swelling of your legs?
- How many pillows do you use at night?
- Do you get short of breath at night?
- How far can you walk without becoming short of breath?
- Have you had any chest pain or palpitations?
- Do you have a cough?

- Do you produce any phlegm?
- Are you taking any tablets that have been prescribed by a doctor?
- Have you felt tired recently?
- Do you have to stop doing things because you become short of breath?
- Do you get better when you rest?

Careful analysis of the answers and the circumstances surrounding them will usually enable a doctor to distinguish between respiratory and cardiac causes of dyspnoea.

Past history

Relevant questions are:

- Have you had any trouble like this before?
- Do you suffer from high blood pressure or any other heart disease?
- Did you have rheumatic fever as a child?
- Do you smoke?

This is not a comprehensive series of questions but those which I actually used to give a wide picture and a high yield of relevant information.

The main causes of heart failure are given in Box 10.1.

Congestive heart failure

This is a mixture of right- and left-sided failure. The signs are:

- congestion of the lungs
- an enlarged heart
- the pulse may be irregular
- there may be abdominal enlargement in severe cases.

There may also be signs of the underlying problem:

- high blood pressure
- valvular heart disease
- chronic obstructive airways disease.

Box 10.1 The main causes of heart failure

1. Left-sided heart failure
    Pressure effects:
    Hypertension
    Aortic stenosis
    Mitral stenosis
    Volume overload:
    Aortic incompetence
    Mitral incompetence
    Patent ductus arteriosus
    Ventricular septal defect

2. Heart muscle disease
    Atherosclerosis
    Cardiomyopathy*
    Endomyocardial fibrosis*

3. Right-heart failure
    Pressure effects
    Pulmonary hypertension
    Chronic obstructive airways disease
      resulting in cor pulmonale
    Pulmonary stenosis
    Multiple pulmonary emboli
    Congenital heart disease
    Volume overload:
    Atrial septal defect
    Tricuspid incompetence

*Rare conditions

Acute left ventricular failure

The main feature is sudden severe shortness of breath—clinically it can appear very similar to an acute attack of bronchospasm. There may be frothy blood-stained sputum, congested lung fields and pulsus alternans.

Mr Greenwood was an accountant, aged 58, who had been admitted to hospital 4 months ago with a coronary thrombosis. He was still seeing the consultant who had reduced his treatment 3 weeks before to allow him to go on holiday. He became progressively short of breath while away and returned home the day before he consulted me. His medication included aspirin and an ACE inhibitor. His answers to my questions indicated that he was very dyspnoeic in hospital. This had slowly

disappeared but had gradually returned during his trip to Spain. He could not sleep without four pillows. He seemed surprised by his deterioration so long after his original trouble.

Having diagnosed congestive cardiac failure it is important to try to discover the underlying cause as this can influence subsequent management.

Who gets heart failure?

A glance at Box 10.1 will show that heart failure is usually a sequel to a pre-existing condition but in general practice it is often the presenting feature. In general practice the most common causes of heart failure are hypertension or ischaemic heart disease. It is a condition of middle-age and beyond but rarely children and babies can also present.

What examination would you now make?

Although the history is very important, the physical signs of heart failure can also help make the diagnosis.

General observations
These are:

- Is the patient dyspnoeic at rest?
- Is there pallor?
- Do the head and neck appear suffused with blood?
- Can the external jugular vein be seen to be engorged?

Systems examination
Heart sounds. There may be a third heart sound and displaced apex beat.

Pulse and blood pressure. The pulse may be faint and irregular or have other characteristics of heart disease. There may be a resting tachycardia. The blood pressure may be very high or low as the condition worsens. Jugular venous pressure is raised. There may be oedema of ankles or sacrum.

Abdomen. A palpable liver or ascites may be detectable.

Respiratory system. Additional breath sounds, moist crepitations or rhonchi, a wheeze, or signs of consolidation at the lung bases may all be present.

It can sometimes be very difficult clinically to differentiate between heart failure and asthma.

In addition to the general impression already mentioned, Mr Greenwood had other physical signs.

His pulse was regular; he was in sinus rhythm. His blood pressure was 110/65 (on the low side?). His external jugular venous pressure was raised up to his ears. He had an enlarged heart with no murmurs. There were moist sounds at the base of both fields. He was clearly in acute heart failure both right- and left-sided.

What tests are available to a GP?

Tests can confirm the clinical impression. ECGs can be difficult to interpret. The first diagnosis depends primarily on your own observations. Available tests include:

1. Weight may have demonstrably increased.
2. The urine can be tested for protein, blood and sugar.
3. An ECG may show signs of a recent or past coronary thrombosis, ventricular enlargement, ischaemia or atrial fibrillation. A normal ECG is unusual in a patient with heart failure.
4. Blood tests may reveal anaemia. Request thyroid function tests.
5. A chest X-ray may show an increased cardiothoracic ratio or pulmonary oedema (giving the appearance known as 'Kerley's B lines').
6. Echocardiography. An echocardiogram is one of the most useful tests—it can determine left ventricle function and also diagnose the cause, e.g. a valve problem. Open access echocardiography is increasingly available for general practitioners. Echocardiography is the investigation of choice for diagnosing heart failure and its cause.

Diagnosis

The diagnosis is reached on the basis of the history, examination and investigations.

Management

The doctor will try to identify the underlying cause but this is only possible in a proportion of cases. The first line of treatment must be based on general principles. Clearly this depends on the speed of onset and the severity but the main treatments are well recognized.

The treatment of heart failure is based on the following principles:

1. Identifying a cause. Echocardiography of value here.

2. Avoidance of drugs worsening/precipitating heart failure, e.g. NSAIDs, tricyclics.
3. Use of loop diuretics to relieve symptoms. In the mildest cases a thiazide may suffice.
4. Consideration of digoxin—may be of use if patient in atrial fibrillation but more controversial if patient is in sinus rhythm.
5. Use of ACE inhibitors. These are the only treatments that significantly improve prognosis. Used with diuretics. Check for contraindications before using and monitor renal function before and during use. Increase dose upwards, to equivalent of 20 mg enalapril a day according to response. ACE inhibitors should be used if left ventricle systolic dysfunction present.
6. Heart failure patients not responding to the above require consultant supervision. The ACE inhibitor may need to be started in hospital if the patient has severe heart failure, is on a high dose diuretic or has renal impairment. Other strategies used by consultants include:

a. use of low dose specific beta-blockers (but general practitioners should avoid beta-blockers in heart failure unless under consultant supervision)
b. nitrates
c. anticoagulation if in atrial fibrillation
d. surgery—including cardiomyoplasty and transplantation.

Mr Greenwood responded well to an increase in diuretics and bed rest. I decided to ask a consultant to make a domiciliary visit.

When to refer to hospital

The decision to refer to hospital is one taken frequently but rarely discussed. It depends on many factors:

1. The knowledge and confidence of the doctor
2. Whether the patient is already under hospital care
3. The wishes of the patient and relatives
4. What back-up services can be provided by the practice in the home
5. The necessity to arrive at a diagnosis
6. The availability of special treatment in hospital, e.g. to start ACE inhibitors
7. Acute left ventricular failure will not permit a leisurely journey to hospital before treatment is commenced.

In general the decision relates to the reason for heart failure and its severity.

On the domiciliary visit the consultant told me that he had seen Mr Greenwood 3 months previously following a severe coronary thrombosis. Hospital investigation showed severe damage superimposed on widespread ischaemic heart disease. He had very poor left ventricular function and moderately impaired renal function.

Clearly the balance was finely tuned. The prognosis was poor. Had he been younger and with no other problems he would have been a candidate for a heart transplant but in this case there was established chronic obstructive airways disease associated with a long history of smoking.

The therapeutic aim was to vasodilate him without increasing his ACE inhibitor and this was achieved by using a long-acting isosorbide mononitrate and increasing still further his frusemide. The treatment was to be monitored by measuring his blood urea and electrolytes at regular intervals. He was still working full time and travelled to work on public transport. The most difficult part of the management was helping him to come to terms with his immediate retirement.

TEACHING POINTS

1. Heart failure is a diagnostic and management challenge. The average general practitioner will have about 20 cases a year.
2. The immediate management can be readily undertaken within general practice but the elucidation of the underlying cause often requires hospital investigations.
3. Long-term management involves extended observations and the patient must be helped to come to terms with the limitations which this condition imposes.

11 A PRESCRIPTION FOR THE PILL

There is no doubt that the combined oral contraceptive pill is the most effective method of contraception (apart from sterilization). It has a pregnancy rate of only 0.1–0.4 per 100 woman-years, compared with 1.5–3.0 for the intrauterine device and 2–3 per 100 woman-years for the progesterone–only pill.

Patients will frequently consult their doctors with problems associated with the pill; some will be questions about how to take them, some will be for real or imagined side-effects and some will be for even broader issues. There are also, of course, specific contraindications to the pill. Those taking the pill require follow-up and a payment is made under the National Health Service for this work. For these reasons the family physician should be an expert in the prescription of the pill and the aftercare this entails. It is wiser to concentrate on knowing a lot about a limited number of pills and to change within this group rather than to try to know a little about each of the numerous alternative pills available.

In this chapter we hope to provide a framework of management for patients on the oral contraceptive pill.

Gillian Page, an 18-year-old girl, comes to you asking to be 'put on the pill'. What initial history would you wish to take?

This request presents less of an ethical problem than if the patient were under 16 years of age, but that is another matter. Age is also important when 35 is approached.

There are broadly three matters on which we might wish to question this girl:

1. The gynaecological history, including details of the last menstrual period in order to exclude pregnancy.

2. Are there any absolute or relative contraindications to her taking the oral contraceptive? Does she suffer from any conditions which might be aggravated by the oral contraceptive? Is she taking any drugs which might interact? Is she a smoker? Is there a family history of thrombosis? Since most family doctors will have a good knowledge of their patient's history, or it will be readily available, this should not take long.

3. Why has she come for contraception now and has she considered other forms of contraception? Has she already used a method of contraception? What does she know about the pill and how it works? Does she know that there are possible side-effects?

Thus, at this initial consultation we are attempting to discover whether this form of contraception is suitable for this girl, and by taking a careful history some of the problems that could arise may be anticipated. The most important question is the third—why does she wish to use the pill? There may be, and usually is, a perfectly sensible and well thought-out reason, but there are a whole variety of reasons why women, especially younger ones, ask for the pill. Some requests for the pill may seem less apparent to the doctor than others: for example, a presentation of dysmenorrhoea may be a covert request for advice on sexual matters and contraception. The doctor has a role as counsellor in these matters and must help the patient to make up her own mind. It is always useful to discuss other possible methods of contraception and the initial discussion should also include a brief account of some of the benefits, risks and common side-effects.

It may be found especially useful to have some form of standard history card or sheet, as in Box 11.1.

At first sight there appears to be a host of absolute and relative contraindications, but many are rare diseases and most others are obvious (Box 11.2). It is worth noting a family history of thromboembolism (in parent or sibling) as some patients have an inherited increased clotting tendency which can be detected by blood tests.

It will be noted that the key to successful pre-

Box 11.1   Sample of a standard history sheet

Age	Marital status
Previous contraception	Previous children

Previous history	*Gynaecological history*
Epilepsy	Cycle length
Diabetes mellitus	Menstrual flow
Cardiovascular disease	Regularity periods
Hypertension	Menarche
Thrombophlebitis	Dysmenorrhoea
Venous thrombosis	Vaginal discharge
Jaundice	Premenstrual history
Migraine/headaches	
Other...	*Personal history*
	Allergies
Family history	Smoking
Diabetes mellitus	Varicose veins
Cardiovascular disease	Contact lenses
	Regular medication

(1) Include any relevant psychosexual history.
(2) Reason for requesting the pill.
(3) Any other special factors.

Box 11.2   Contraindications to the contraceptive pill

1. *Absolute contraindications to the combined pill*
Known or suspected pregnancy
Hydatidiform mole
Hormone dependent tumours
Impaired liver function
Thromboembolic disorders (including deep vein thrombosis, pulmonary embolism, cerebrovascular accident, myocardial infarction, transient ischaemic attacks)
Severe hypertension
Migraine with focal symptoms
Any condition of the circulatory system predisposing to thromboembolism (including atrial fibrillation)
Pituitary disease
Porphyria
Sickle cell anaemia
Undiagnosed irregular genital tract bleeding
Long-term immobilization

Four weeks prior to elective major surgery
Chronic pancreatitis

2. *Relative contraindications to the combined pill*
In these cases balance the risks of pregnancy: monitor closely and choose pills with care
Oligo- or amenorrhoea in the young. Risk that the pill may affect subsequent ovulation
Fibroids may enlarge with the pill
Mild to moderate hypertension. The pill may cause it or worsen it
Obesity. Increases the risks of the pill
Smoking. Increases the risks of the pill
Migraine. May appear for the first time. May be aggravated by the pill
Diabetes mellitus. Combined pills reduce glucose tolerance; drug dose may need to be adjusted
Hyperlipidaemia
Severe depression
Epilepsy
Lactation; suppressed but progestogen-only pills may be used
Contact lenses may be found uncomfortable due to corneal oedema
Occasionally varicose veins are aggravated

3. *Notes on cancer and the combined pill*
The combined pill is known to protect against ovarian and endometrial cancer. There may be a link between use of oral contraceptives and breast cancer but more research is required and the increased risk is likely to be small

scription lies in the assessment of risk factors, especially *age, weight, smoking, high blood pressure, diabetes mellitus*. While one risk factor may be acceptable, two or more may not.

Drug interactions

The effectiveness of the pill can be reduced by drugs and the interference is usually signalled by spotting or breakthrough bleeding. Doctors should therefore warn the patient, especially with regard to antibiotics given for infections while the patient is taking the pill.

Interactions which can reduce effectiveness include

antibiotics (e.g. ampicillin), tranquillizers and anti-convulsants.

Oral contraceptives may potentiate the effect of corticosteroids.

Oral contraceptives may decrease the effects of anti-coagulants and insulin.

Which pill would you prescribe for this patient and how would you manage any side-effects?

There are numerous types of oral contraceptives to choose from. In recent years there have been several changes in the combined pill formulations available. Recent studies have suggested that the so-called 'third-generation' pills containing desogestrel and gestodene have a higher risk of thromboembolism than the 'second-generation' pills. Current advice for most women would be to start on one of these 'second-generation' pills not containing gestodene or deso-gestrel, e.g. Microgynon or Ovranette. Progestogen-only pills (e.g. Noriday, Neogest) should be used in lactating women, those over 35 who smoke, women with diabetes mellitus and those who have had severe oestrogen effects previously.

It is still possible to grade pills into a table of in-creasing progestogen (Table 11.1). Note that pills containing 50 µg of oestrogen should be reserved for use only where absorption is likely to be a problem or there are possible drug interactions.

Table 11.1 A list of increasing progestogen levels

Preparation	Oestrogen/progestogen	
Norethisterone pills		
Norimin	Ethinyloestradiol	35 µg
	Norethisterone	1 mg
Synphase (a phasic pill)	Ethinyloestradiol	35 µg
	Norethisterone	0.5 mg (7 tabs) 1 mg
		(9 tabs) 0.5 mg (5 tabs)
Brevinor	Ethinyloestradiol	35 µg
	Norethisterone	0.5 mg
Levonorgestrel pills		
Eugynon 30	Ethinyloestradiol	30 µg
	Levonorgestrel	250 µg
Microgynon 30	Ethinyloestradiol	30 µg
	Levonorgestrel	150 µg
Logynon (a phasic pill)	Ethinyloestradiol	30 µg
	Levonorgestrel	50 µg (6 tabs)
		75 µg (5 tabs)
		125 µg (10 tabs)

Table 11.2 Side-effects of the contraceptive pill

May be associated with oestrogen excess	May be associated with progestogen excess
Nausea and vomiting	Acne, greasy hair
Migraine and headaches	Increased appetite
Thromboembolic disease	Decreased libido
Chloasma	Dry vagina
Mucoid vaginal discharge	

Table 11.2 lists side-effects that may be associated with oestrogen and progestogen excess.

Side-effects

The following are some of the major and common minor side-effects that occur with the pill.

1. Breakthrough bleeding (BTB). Bleeding or spotting is common in the first two cycles, particularly with low dose pills. Check that the BTB was not caused by diarrhoea interfering with absorption, drug interactions or a missed pill. If BTB persists try a pill with increased progestogen.

2. Amenorrhoea or oligomenorrhoea. Absent menstruation on the pill-free days is usually a feature of the low dose pills in the first few cycles. Having excluded pregnancy this need not be an undue worry.

3. Nausea. One of the most common of all re-ported side-effects is nausea and even vomiting. Fortunately after the first few cycles these symptoms usually regress. Nausea can be reduced by taking the pill at night, preferably with food.

4. Headache. If migraine appears for the first time or is worsened by the pill it should be stopped. Stop the pill if headaches are associated with any other visual, motor or sensory symptoms. Rarely it may be the first sign of developing hypertension.

5. Cervical erosions. The so-called cervical 'erosion' is commonly seen in pill users. Beware of ascribing symptoms to them—the majority are asymptomatic and best ignored.

6. Depression. Depression is easily ascribed to the pill, when the root cause may be personal problems unrelated to any hormone. There does however seem to be a group of women who do get depressed with the pill and pyridoxine deficiency has been suggested as the mechanism. A trial of a pill with a different progestogen might be helpful.

7. Hypertension. This is rarely severe and seems to be largely reversible, returning to normal about 3 months after stopping the pill. Hypertension can occur at any stage and is especially prevalent in those with a family history of hypertension. The incidence of hypertension is said to be less than 1% in the first year, but after 5 years' usage it rises to more than 1 in 40. A small rise in blood pressure may be managed by changing to a lower-dose pill with careful monitoring. Malignant hypertension can develop with the pill. In general if the diastolic BP rises by more than 15 mmHg or to above a value of 90 mmHg the pill should be stopped. Take into account the presence or absence of other risk factors, especially age, weight and smoking.

8. Gallbladder disease. The incidence of cholelithiasis and cholecystitis is higher in pill users.

9. Post-pill amenorrhoea. One golden rule— exclude pregnancy first. The majority will menstruate. If there is still no menstruation after 6 months, refer to a gynaecologist—drugs may be needed, as may investigation to exclude a prolactin-secreting pituitary adenoma. The need to conceive often determines the referral.

10. Candidiasis. Recent studies do not tend to support the suggestion that candidiasis is much more common on the pill, but it may be more resistant to treatment and may need a short term off the pill.

A knowledge of the above enables sensible changes to be made by decreasing and increasing the relative hormonal composition of the pill used. A few major risks are dealt with later.

Prescribing in special situations

Post partum
During the first 6 months after delivery, contraception is not required if:

1. the infant is fed exclusively with the mother's own breast milk, *and*
2. she remains amenorrhoeic.

The risk of pregnancy exists:

1. as soon as these conditions do not exist, or
2. she stops providing all the baby's nutritional needs, or
3. she starts menstruating, or
4. is 6 months post partum.

In the perimenopausal period
Risk of cardiovascular disease and breast cancer increases as women approach the menopause. Their assessment is the same as for younger women. Smoking has a more pronounced effect on the risk of cardiovascular disease in older women. Perimenopausal women who wish to use combined oral contraceptives must give up smoking. Non-smoking perimenopausal women can use combined oral contraceptives through their menopause.

Epilepsy
Combined oral contraceptives reduce the effectiveness of enzyme-inducing antiepileptic drugs such as phenytoin and carbamazepine. Women on these drugs should be switched to antiepileptic drugs that do not interfere with the metabolism of combined oral contraceptives (alternatively, some doctors prescribe higher oestrogen dose preparations).

Liver disease
There is limited information but long term use may be associated with rare liver conditions such as cholestasis, benign hepatocellular carcinoma and benign liver tumours. Combined oral contraceptives are contraindicated in women with hepatic disease but can be used in those with a history of viral hepatitis, provided their liver enzyme tests are normal.

Sickle cell disease
There is an increased risk of thrombosis in those with this disease; but pregnancy is also particularly hazardous. There is no contraindication for those with sickle cell trait.

Having taken a history and prescribed the pill, what examination would you make and how would you follow up the patient?

The follow-up should focus on measuring the blood pressure, assessing cardiovascular risk status and advising on side-effects and any specific problems. Routine weighing and urine testing is not worthwhile. The follow-up consultations are a good chance to: (1) educate re breast self-examination; (2) ensure the patient is immune to rubella; (3) discourage smoking; (4) reinforce the value of cervical cytology screening.

Fear of a vaginal examination deters many women from seeking advice on family planning and routine vaginal examination is unnecessary unless the gynae-cological history demands it or pregnancy is suspected. The first cervical smear should be carried out within 1 or 2 years of the start of sexual activity, repeated after 1 year to exclude false negatives and then re-peated at 3–5 yearly intervals. Patients vary: with a nervous 17-year-old just about to start the pill, vaginal examination is unnecessary and smears can probably be left until a later date; with a 30-year-old multi-parous patient an early smear will be more acceptable.

Suggested follow-up

- Initial consultation: BP. Smear (if not done at this visit, do on follow-up visit).
- 3 months later: BP. Ask about cycle control/side-effects. Is she happy with her pill?
- 6 months from initial consultation: BP. First smear if not done at initial visit, or postpone if indicated (see above).
- Every 6 months thereafter: At each visit, BP. Any side-effects? Any new cardiovascular risk factors? Every 3 years: cervical smear.

What instructions would you give Ms Page about taking the pill?

This is every bit as important as the rest of the consul-tation because failure to explain a few simple details could well lead to dissatisfaction, non-compliance or even pregnancy. Do not assume that the patient will read the leaflet in the packet!

1. All the newer pills start on the first day of menstruation. With a pill starting on the first day of menstruation additional contraception is not required, but it will be required (for 14 days) when the pill is started on the fifth day.

2. Warn the patient of a few of the common minor problems that may occur and reassure her that they usually disappear after the early cycles. The advice must include a mention of breakthrough bleeding as this particularly alarms the patient.

3. Advice on factors reducing protection with the combined pill is important. Tell the patient:
   a. that if she forgets to take a pill she should take the next one within 12 hours or protection is reduced. If more than 12 hours have passed without a pill, she should continue the packet

but take additional precautions for the next 7 days. The Family Planning Association advise that if a pill is missed and the patient has less than 7 pills left in the packet, the next packet of pills should be started without a break (i.e. no pill-free interval).
   b. that diarrhoea and vomiting reduce the effectiveness; she should continue the packet and take extra precautions as outlined in (a) above.
   c. that she should be aware of drug interactions; breakthrough bleeding may be a sign that effectiveness is reduced.
   d. to remember to mention that she is on the pill if she is hospitalized for any reason.

The instructions above will, of course, differ with the progestogen-only pill.

What are the major risks of the combined pill?

The major risks of the pill have now been assessed in many classical studies, including those by Vessey and Doll in the late 1960s, the prospective study by the Royal College of General Practitioners in Britain, and the Walnut Creek study and the Boston Colla-borative Drug Surveillance Programme in the United States. The serious risks include:

1. cardiovascular: thromboembolism, myocardial infarction, hypertension, cerebrovascular disease (including subarachnoid haemorrhage)
2. gallbladder and liver disease.

Hepatocellular adenoma may be more common with high-dose pills used over several years (see Box 11.2 for other associations of the pill and cancer). The overall risk of the pill is low, with about 5 deaths for every 100 000 users under 35 years of age. This figure rises sixfold for those over 35. For patients over 35 the use of the combined pill cannot be re-commended if other risk factors, such as smoking, are present. However, healthy non-smoking women can continue a low dose combined pill until the menopause.

The pill must be stopped if any of the following occur:

1. migraine if severe, with focal features or it is the patient's first attack
2. deep vein thrombosis or pulmonary embolism

3. pregnancy
4. serious hypertension (see before)
5. jaundice
6. other circulatory conditions, e.g. myocardial
   infarction
7. before operation or before prolonged immobility
   in bed.

TEACHING POINTS

1. The combined oral contraceptive pill is the most highly effective method of contraception apart from sterilization.
2. General practitioners should be experts in contraception and be knowledgeable about the contraindications, drug interactions, side-effects and prescription of the oral contraceptive pills available.
3. When assessing any patient for the contraceptive pill remember the risk factors, including weight, smoking and blood pressure.
4. There should be a planned follow-up of patients, and the opportunity for health education should not be missed.
5. When the patient is starting the oral contraceptive pill, spend time explaining not only how to use it but also factors that reduce protection and common minor problems.

12 HORMONE REPLACEMENT THERAPY

The 'menopause' is the term used for the cessation of menstruation in women. The average age at which it occurs is 51; 5% of women stop having periods before the age of 45 and 5% continue beyond the age of 55. As the definition is the last menstrual period it can only be diagnosed in retrospect. This pattern has not changed since the nineteenth century but life expectancy has. It is now 82–83 years. Nine out of ten women reach the menopause and the average woman spends one-third of her life in the postmenopausal state. In the United Kingdom there are some 10 million postmenopausal women, forming 18% of the total population.

Postmenopausal women lose 15% of bone mass within 5 years of the menopause and continue at an annual rate of 0.6% thereafter. Between one-third and one one half of non-treated women will have an osteoporotic fracture in later life.

During the climacteric a similar proportion (one-third to one half) of women will suffer from some form of psychological complaint. The incidence of cardio-vascular disease doubles within 20 years in those who have an oophorectomy, or a premature menopause. Oestrogens reduce this risk to normal.

Prescription of hormone replacement therapy (HRT) has increased substantially in recent years, due in part to the recognition of its benefits not only in preventing osteoporosis but in reducing the risk of heart attacks. It is now widely requested by patients.

Mrs Dorset, a woman in her late 40s who works as a home-help, plonked herself down opposite me and somewhat hurriedly said: 'I've come to ask you about this hormone treatment. Some say it's good, some say it's bad, so I thought I would come and see what you have to say.'

It is a little unusual to be asked such an open-ended question at the beginning of the consultation so it may be wise to pause for a moment to consider the situation.

The presentation suggests that Mrs Dorset may feel flustered. Why? Is she embarrassed or really only in a hurry? Is she being pressurized by her relatives and friends or is this a straightforward question?

One approach would be to say 'Well I'd like to help you but it's a big topic. What made you think of coming to see me today?' It turned out that she mentioned some of her uncomfortable symptoms to several friends who gave a variety of unhelpful and conflicting answers.

What are the most important questions to answer even if they are not always asked?

1. Will it make me feel better?
2. Should I take it?
3. Is it safe?
4. Does it have side-effects?
5. How long should I take it for?

Will it make me feel better?

The acute symptoms of oestrogen deficiency, typically hot flushes and night sweats, are experienced by approximately 75% of menopausal women. One-quarter do not suffer at all.

Box 12.1 lists the main menopausal symptoms and HRT will certainly relieve many of these. Apart from symptom relief, there are long-term benefits in the prevention of cardiovascular disease and osteoporosis.

Our patients should be given a balanced view of the current state of medical opinion and helped to come to their own decision.

What are the benefits and disadvantages?

Box 12.2 lists the benefits and disadvantages of HRT. Note that with continuous combined HRT the patient may not now need regular periods if she is to use HRT.

Box 12.1 List of menopausal symptoms

- *Neuroendocrine*
  Hot flushes
  Night sweats
  Insomnia
  Mood changes
  Depression
  Anxiety
  Irritability
  Loss of memory
  Poor concentration
  Nervousness

- *Genital tract*
  Vaginal dryness
  Dyspareunia
  Loss of libido
  Urinary frequency
  Urgency
  Stress incontinence

- *Cardiovascular*
  Palpitations

- *Miscellaneous*
  Joint/muscle aches
  Dry skin
  Brittle nails/hair
  Parasthesiae
  Fatigue/lethargy

Box 12.2 The benefits and disadvantages of HRT

- *Benefits*
  Relief of climacteric symptoms
  Risk of coronary heart disease reduced by
  50%
  Major reduction in the risk of developing
  osteoporosis
  Benefit in Alzheimer's disease
  Reduction in rate of fatal colonic cancer

- *Disadvantages*
  Return of menses (not a problem with some
  of the newer HRT preparations)
  Possible 35% increase risk of breast cancer
  (women on HRT > 10 years)
  Side-effects of treatment

What are the contraindications to HRT?

These are listed in Box 12.3.

Is is safe and does it have side-effects?

The major long-term hazard of unopposed oestrogens is the effect on the endometrium and the increased risk of endometrial carcinoma in those who have not had a hysterectomy.

The incidence of endometrial hyperplasia and carcinoma has been significantly reduced by the addition of a progestogen for 12 days each month. We now know there is a slight increased risk of breast cancer with HRT use. The risk is related to duration of use, increasing the risk by 2.3% for each year of use. Family history of breast cancer does not alter the HRT-associated risk. The excess risk becomes negligible after 5 years of stopping HRT.

Side-effects of treatment occur in approximately 5% and include nausea, breast tenderness, leg cramps, headache and weight gain. These problems may be improved by using a smaller dose of oestrogen or using an alternative route such as transdermal patches. The problems specific to transdermal oestrogen include erythema on the site of the patch and irritation.

Box 12.3 Contraindications to hormone replacement therapy

- *Absolute contraindications*
  A current oestrogen-dependent tumour
  (breast, genital tract)
  Undiagnosed vaginal bleeding
  Active thromboembolic disease
  Severe active liver disease

  Note: consider other risk factors.
  Hypertension should be controlled before
  starting HRT. Since HRT is of benefit in
  protecting from heart disease, the presence
  of heart disease is not a contraindication.

- *Relative contraindications*
  Diabetes
  Gallstones
  Fibroids
  Endometriosis
  Otosclerosis
  Malignant melanoma

Breakthrough bleeding is an indication for hysteroscopy. There may also be premenstrual syndrome-like problems, e.g. headaches, bloating, fluid retention and acne, which are progestogen related. You can try changing the progestogen.

How long can I take it for?

Duration of treatment is largely determined by the indications of commencing treatment. For the majority of women the indication is the relief of flushes and they are likely to require it for 2 to 5 years on average. However, if it is to be used to prevent loss of bone mass then the patient is likely to require continuous treatment for 10 to 15 years. Up to 10 years of treatment will reduce risk of fractured neck of femur by 40–45%. After 10 years the incidence of breast cancer rises, so the current best advice is to use HRT for 10 years and reassess the continuing need then. Clearly before embarking on long-term therapy, the benefits of treatment must be weighed against the disadvantages.

What forms of treatment are there?

The main routes are:

1. Oral route. This is the most commonly used one and is very convenient for those who do not object to taking tablets and are reasonably compliant. Contraindications for this route are:
   a. Those predisposed to hypertension. In hypertension they may increase the renin substrate production. These effects are mediated via a first pass metabolic affect on the liver and a non-oral route administration avoiding such hepatic effects is appropriate.
   b. They should not be given to women with a history of clotting disorders because antithrombin free activity may be depressed.

In patients with a uterus the preparation must contain progesterone for 10–14 days per month.

2. Vaginal gels and creams, e.g. dienoestrol cream.

3. Subcutaneous implants (50–100 mg of oestradiol every 6 months).

4. Transdermal patches. The transdermal route delivers oestrogen into the systemic, not the portal circulation. This route has a theoretical advantage for patients with hypertension and cardiovascular disease (or a high risk of such). The oestrodial patch must be combined with oral progesterone in those women who have not had a hysterectomy. If the uterus is present the patient must take progesterone for 10–14 days per month

5. Continuous combined HRT has now become available and consists of a daily dose of oestrogen and progesterone. After a few months the patient may become amenorrhoeic—giving the advantages of HRT without periods! Examples include Climesse, Evorel Conti, Kliofem and Premique.

A PLAN FOR MANAGING THE MENOPAUSE

The doctor or practice nurse should ask him or herself these questions about the patient.

1. Why now?
2. What symptons do you have that will benefit?
3. What is your present state of knowledge of HRT?
4. Do I know the risks and benefits?
5. Have I asked about her lifestyle?
6. Can we make the decision to proceed?
7. Am I able to give follow-up care?
8. Do I know when to review and how often?
9. Do I know when to recommend it should stop?
10. Have I got a good booklet with the right information?

Management

Increasingly hormone replacement therapy is one of the key topics in a 'well person' examination. Practice nurses are now managing most of the patients established on HRT.

1. The initial consultation

History. Are there positive symptoms of oestrogen deficiency (Box 12.1)? Date of LMP? Any bleeding (postmenopausal bleeding needs investigating)? Hysterectomy? Were ovaries removed? Are there any osteoporosis risk factors present? Does she want to take hormones? Discuss contraception. Contraception is required for 1 year after the last menstrual period if the patient is aged over 50 or 2 years after the last menstrual period if the patient is under age 50. Are there any contraindications to HRT?

Examination. Are there any breast lumps? Pelvic masses on PV examination? BP and cardiovascular risk factors? Use a urine dipstick for proteinuria and glycosuria.

Investigations if indicated. Smear; Mammogram. A blood test for FSH can confirm ovarian failure if there is any diagnostic doubt.

2. Review consultations

Practice nurse every 6 months, doctor every 2 years. At each visit:

1. Ask about problems with HRT and menstrual bleeding patterns.
2. Check weight, self-examination of breasts, date of last smear, BP (refer to general practitioner if ≥100 mmHg diastolic).

3. Offer general advice about the menopause (with a leaflet), osteoporosis and coronary heart disease prevention.

TEACHING POINTS

1. Attitudes to hormone replacement have changed over the years.
2. There is a clear advantage to some patients.
3. The introduction of well person clinics offers an opportunity to follow patients in a systematic way.

13 HAY FEVER

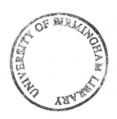

Hay fever is a common illness and most of us know someone with the problem. The prevalence in general practice is over 10% of the population and the incidence is increasing. It has a peak incidence in the ages 5–30, being most common in the first half of this range. In many of the patients there will be a family history of atopic illness (hay fever, asthma, eczema) and the hay fever itself may be associated with asthma (about a third of cases have so-called 'pollen asthma'), eczema, perennial rhinitis or urticaria.

The most characteristic feature of hay fever, which may be regarded as a type I hypersensitivity to the allergen pollen, is its seasonal nature. In England, when caused by the inhalation of grass pollen, it tends to start dramatically in late May or early June, lasting through June and July (Fig. 13.1). In much rarer cases where tree pollen is indicated it may occur in April or May; mould spores have more variable peaks and are said to be responsible for hay fever in late summer and early autumn. There are geographical variations in that the grass pollen season, for example, occurs slightly later in the north of England than in the south.

A young law student, Peter Green, new to the Practice, consulted recently. He had had numerous coughs and colds as a child, and from the age of 10 had had severe bouts of sneezing, rhinorrhoea and eye soreness every year. This time it was clearly worse. His eyes were red, watering and sore. He had a dry cough which at night was associated with some wheezing. He had taken some antihistamine tablets that he had at home to no avail, and he had also used a Rynacrom nasal spray previously prescribed. He apologized for attending but said he needed 'something strong' as he was due to take an important exam in a few days and could not concentrate in his present condition.

What are the main symptoms of hay fever and what are the main points in the history to ask about if you suspect hay fever?

The diagnosis is made on the basis of the clinical and family history of symptoms. There are three sites commonly affected in hay fever due to allergy to pollen.

1. Nasal symptoms. The most common symptoms, usually occurring together, are sneezing, rhinorrhoea (a copious clear water discharge from the nose), itching of the nose and bilateral blockage of the nasal passages. The nasal mucosa changes to a pale colour with a bluish tinge, and as oedema increases polyp-

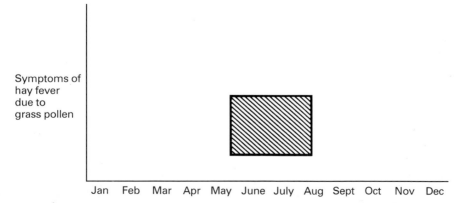

Fig. 13.1 The hay fever season due to grass pollen.

like projections may develop. An auriscope with a nasal speculum can be used to inspect the inside of the nose, as a polyp should be considered in anyone with persistent nasal symptoms.

2. Ocular symptoms. There is usually a conjunctivitis with redness, itching and watering of the eyes.

3. Chest symptoms. Some patients may complain of chest tightness, cough or wheeze, or shortness of breath.

A few patients complain of a 'tickling' sensation at the back of the throat.

With typical symptoms such as these occurring in the pollen season there should be little problem in diagnosis. Occasionally one symptom will be more prominent and it may present as a resistant 'cold' or stuffy nose. In some patients wheezing is the most prominent symptom.

We may look at the history to bring out a few interesting points.

1. Age. The majority of cases occur before puberty and only 10% commence after the age of 30. It is said that the younger the presentation the more likely the history of other atopic conditions.

2. Symptoms and natural history. The symptoms may be worse in the morning (when more pollen is released), relieved during rainy spells and exacerbated by exposure, e.g. a walk in the country. The seasonal incidence of late May to mid-July, typical of grass pollen allergy in the south of England, is also helpful in diagnosis. The pollen count during the season is often publicized by the media. Thus in the history enquire about (a) seasonal and diurnal variation, (b) relation to weather, (c) relation to exposure to environment, e.g. worse indoors or outdoors.

Hay fever is a recurrent illness; however, after several seasons, usually from 5 to 15, the symptoms do abate, so it does resolve naturally in the end.

3. Previous/present history of allergic conditions. Hay fever is one of a spectrum of allergic conditions, and sufferers may have or have had associated problems, such as asthma, urticaria, eczema, etc.

4. Family history. Ask for a family history of allergic conditions (hay fever, asthma, eczema, perennial rhinitis, urticaria). The more positive a family history and the more allergic the patient, the more difficult to control and the more chronic the hay fever is likely to be. No history is of course complete without asking patients about self-medication and you may well be surprised by the answers!

What is the differential diagnosis of hay fever, and what other environmental agents are there?

This patient's symptoms are consistent with hay fever, but this is a convenient point to look at some common allergies. In fact, nocturnal cough and wheezing is more common in house dust mite allergy than in hay fever, but in house dust mite allergy the symptoms are not more prominent in the May-June-July period.

Humans are subject to a wide range of allergies and these other allergens must be considered when atypical histories are obtained. In particular, perennial rather than seasonal symptoms are explained by allergies such as house dust, house dust mite, animal danders and foods. It is frequently found that a patient is sensitive to multiple allergens.

HOUSE DUST MITE ALLERGY

The house dust mite is one of the most common allergens to cause problems. The mite, *Dermatophagoides pteronyssinus*, feeds on shed human skin scales. It thrives in warmth and humidity and no house is free from it. It may cause a perennial wheeze and chronic rhinitis and should be considered in all patients with a chronic 'stuffy nose'. The mite and its products are usually wafted into the air on bedmaking and thus symptoms occur most at night, on waking and in the bedroom. The symptoms may be at their height in the autumn, coinciding with maximum proliferation of the mite. The wheezing and rhinitis can be treated along similar lines as hay fever (see below).

Advice is most important and should include:

1. regular vacuum cleaning of mattress, floor, etc.
2. removing feather pillows and eiderdowns, replacing them with those having synthetic fillings
3. enclosing the mattress in a plastic cover
4. thorough cleaning of carpets, curtains, etc.
5. changing and washing bed linen frequently.

The differentiation of the two allergies should thus be easy (Table 13.1).

Before being totally diverted you may wish to revise your knowledge of the diagnosis of a chronic stuffy nose. All rhinitis is not hay fever or house dust mite allergy. Recurrent sinusitis with upper respiratory tract infection is one possibility. Vasomotor rhinitis can

Table 13.1 Differentiating between pollen and house dust mite allergies

	Pollen	House dust mite
Symptoms	Rhinorrhoea Conjuctivitis	Mainly rhinitis and wheeze
Symptoms occur	Seasonally	Perennially
Symptoms more severely	Outdoors	Indoors, bedroom
Time of day	Often morning	Mostly nocturnal in bedroom

simulate hay fever—here the rhinitis changes with humidity and temperature. Occupational exposure to some agents, e.g. chrome, is a rare cause. Nasal obstruction due to a polyp or foreign body can occur and this may be a cause of a persistent stuffy nose in a patient where conventional therapy has failed; hence our advice to inspect the nose. Lastly, the prolonged use of vasoconstrictor decongestant drops can be associated with a chronic stuffy nose.

Causes of a stuffy nose can therefore be summarized thus:

- infection (viral, bacterial, sinusitis)
- allergy (hay fever, house dust mite)
- vasomotor rhinitis
- obstruction (polyp, foreign body, deviated septum)
- medication.

Lastly, we can list the major allergens to which humans are susceptible. Food allergy is a big subject we shall not discuss here. In a patient with atypical symptoms, always ask about pets and drugs, aspirin for example.

SOME MAJOR ALLERGENS

1. pollens
   grass: timothy (the most allergenic), cocksfoot, meadow fescue, rye grass
   tree: birch, hazel, poplar
   flowers and shrubs: e.g. nettle, plantain
2. fungi
3. house dust mite
4. moulds
5. pets: cats, rabbits, dogs
6. foods, including cows' milk protein
7. drugs, e.g. aspirin.

How would you have treated this patient?

He has said that he has to sit an important examination in a few days' time and clearly he is in no fit state to take it. I had no qualms about prescribing steroids. There are two alternatives, injection or an oral course.

1. Injection. Intramuscular injection of corticosteroid is not now recommended. It has been used in the past but, while a single injection may relieve hay fever symptoms throughout a season, any side-effects are difficult to reverse. There is a high risk of adrenal suppression, lasting for well over a month.

2. Oral course. Oral corticosteroids are an option in severe cases failing to respond to other treatment. A short course (e.g. 20 mg prednisolone for 5 days) is useful to treat the patient at times of important life events. It avoids the need for injection, is more flexible, can be stopped without fear, and has no side-effects such as muscle wasting at the site of injection.

The proper and supervised use of steroids for short courses in severe sufferers is wholly justified.

I gave my patient an oral course of prednisolone to tide him over the examination.

What other additional or alternative therapies are there for hay fever?

1. Advice

- Listen to pollen forecast in the media. If count is high:
  keep windows and doors closed
  minimize time spent outdoors
  shower and wash hair on return
- Keep car windows and vents shut
- Consider installing a car pollen filter
- Avoid cutting grass, picnics, camping
- Wear glasses or sunglasses
- Before evening (as air cools), bring in washing and close bedroom windows
- Avoid irritants such as tobacco smoke.

2. Antihistamines. For patients with mild hay fever antihistamines may be all that is required. Antihistamines can relieve the symptoms of itching, sneezing and rhinorrhoea but not the symptoms of nasal blockage. Use the newer non-sedating antihistamines. Patients should still be warned about driving and operating machinery. Avoid their use in pregnancy and remember the possibility of drug interactions.

Side-effects, including arrhythmias, can occur with certain antihistamines (terfenadine and astemizole) and we now use the newer agents like loratadine, cetirizine and fexofenadine. Check what medication the patient has already taken before prescribing.

3. *Symptomatic relief.* **Ocular:** dark glasses help. Sodium cromoglycate 2% drops (Opticrom) is the treatment of choice here but they must be used regularly and their prophylactic role explained to the patient. Steroid drops are an alternative but general practitioners would be unwise to use them, considering the potential damage they may cause, for allergic conjunctivitis due to hay fever. **Nasal:** vasoconstrictor nose drops are to be avoided—rebound symptoms may occur when they are stopped. There are other nasal preparations. Sodium cromoglycate can be administered as a nasal spray (Rynacrom) but it needs to be given four times a day. Intranasal steroid preparations are generally more effective, and continuous therapy can render a dramatic improvement. The local steroids, budesonide, fluticasone, mometasone and triamcinolone, are examples; with all, reduce the dose to the minimum. Topical steroids may take several days before their effect is noticed by the patient. Patients should be warned about the delayed onset of action. Check compliance, as failure to take nasal sprays continuously is a common reason for poor symptom control. Unlike antihistamines intranasal steroids relieve the nasal obstruction as well as other symptoms. Some can be given once daily. Side-effects are generally mild, e.g. nasal irritation or minor bleeding. In those who experienced severe symptoms in the previous year, treatment should be started about 3 weeks before the hay fever season begins. A good policy to monitor usage. **Chest:** pollen asthma is treated with bronchodilators for the acute phase and sodium cromoglycate (Intal) or inhaled steroid as a preventative measure.

Start with a good assessment; how severe are the symptoms and which ones are troubling the patient most? Start with simple preparations such as antihistamines plus local agents. For most patients with moderate hay fever a topical nasal spray will be required.

Peter said he had heard of courses of injections which make you less sensitive to pollen and asked if he could have them straight away.

How would you have responded?

He was referring to desensitization procedures; in these, by using courses of subcutaneous injections of the allergen to which the patient is sensitive, a blocking antibody is produced and the patient's tolerance of the allergen increased. The injections are pre-seasonal and, while improvement may occur after one pre-seasonal course usually about three consecutive years of treatment are needed for good effect. Deaths from anaphylactic shock have occurred with these desensitizing vaccines and the Committee on Safety of Medicines has recommended that they should be given only where full facilities for cardiorespiratory resuscitation exist. The defence organisation would find it difficult to defend a doctor performing these desensitizations in other circumstances and thus effectively desensitization is now solely a hospital procedure.

The problem can quite easily be explained to Peter, perhaps adding that today's treatments are in any case usually effective in controlling symptoms.

TEACHING POINTS

1. Hay fever due to grass pollen is seasonal; in England, starting in late May and lasting through June and July.
2. The main symptoms are nasal and ocular.
3. Hay fever is not the only cause of nasal symptoms. Allergy to the house dust mite should be considered in all patients with a chronic stuffy nose.
4. In mild hay fever start treatment with simple preparations.
5. Do not be afraid of using short courses of steroids for hay fever if the situation demands it.
6. Desensitization is now effectively a hospital procedure.

14 DEPRESSION

Anxiety and depression are common words and do not have an exclusively medical meaning. If anxiety is used to describe the human response to a threat of injury, psychological or physical, real or imagined, depression is the response to loss in the same broad categories. It is a challenge for the doctor to recognize the existence of depression in patients, to try to identify its origin and to assess whether a therapeutic response will help and, if so, in what form.

The shock which awaits the newcomer to primary care is considerable and it will take time to adjust to the multifaceted presentation of human response to the experience of life. How true it is that 'Deception and hypocrisy are two very human strategies for dealing with the complexities of life.'

It is also important to remember that patients presenting with anxiety may also have an underlying depression.

There are many estimates of the prevalence of depression, but as no definition is agreed it is difficult to place much reliance on the figures. In one account, depression was the second most common diagnosis made; anxiety was placed fifth. The current situation is summarized by the following statement. About 10% of all patients consulting a doctor are suffering from some form of clinically recognizable depression. Nine out of ten of these patients are treated by their own general practitioner; more than half of them have so-called masked depression.

The patient presenting to a doctor complaining of feeling depressed or with symptoms which suggest a depression requires an appropriate response. First, stress the following points:

- It is a common illness.
- There are good treatments with successful outcomes.
- There is a biochemical basis for the condition.
- It need not be a stigma.
- Antidepressant tablets are not addictive.

Secondly, an assessment must be made of the severity of the condition and this will largely determine the management. The range of symptoms is wide; the response can range from sympathy and an opportunity to talk, through drug therapy, to urgent admission to hospital. Life events are frequently associated with such presentations and attempts have been made to grade these. Box 14.1 shows typical life events in order of importance.

As well as these so-called life crises, a number of factors are recognized as predisposing to depression and can be elicited in a history. These are:

1. a long history of depression
2. a manic-depressive illness
3. a severe attack of depression
4. more than one episode continuing for 2 weeks.

There are also a number of situations which render the patient much more vulnerable; the following are examples:

1. loss of a mother before the age of 11
2. cancer in the family
3. women with three or more children under 14
4. postnatal period
5. bereavement, especially widows with no family
6. the elderly
7. poor diet
8. social isolation.

Box 14.1 Significant life events in order of importance

1. Death of a loved one—child, spouse, relative
2. Divorce
3. Loss of job
4. Breakdown of relationships
5. Moving house
6. Adverse financial circumstances, etc.
7. Chronic painful physical illness

Albert Ridgeway, a patient aged 58, is an ex-miner in receipt of an invalidity pension for pneumoconiosis. He is being treated for hypertension and, at his routine monthly appointment, complains of headaches. On further questioning he describes them as a feeling of pressure and they have made him feel low and he is worried about them.

What questions would you ask?

A useful framework for questions relevant to any pain is: the site, the quality of the pain (is it stabbing, boring, etc?), its intensity, the exact time sequence, associated symptoms (such as sweating, vomiting, etc.), secondary features (such as fainting, palpitations, diarrhoea, or any other symptom), and finally the patient's attitude and thoughts about the pain.

The headaches are frontal, and feel like a tight band. There are no associated symptoms. He is not sleeping and is worried in case he has a brain tumour. On examination there was no local tenderness. His blood pressure was well controlled. There had been no change of treatment recently. His sleep pattern should now be elucidated. He had no difficulty in getting off to sleep but wakes at about 4 a.m. At this time he felt awful and was convinced that he had a brain tumour. He has tried aspirin and codeine for his headaches without relief.

The story is now suggestive of a depressive episode. A brief glance at Table 14.1 will show the main symptoms of anxiety and depression. Further details can be obtained by studying the various rating scales mentioned in the latter part of this chapter. A knowledge of these will enable the appropriate questions to be asked.

With further questioning you discover that his mother did indeed die before he was 11, and that recently his brother-in-law died of cancer. He has lost all his interest in his home and his hobbies. He feels unworthy of his family and is convinced that he has a brain tumour.

How would you assess whether he is suicidal?

Direct questioning is the only available method. Most people prefer to talk about bodily symptoms because they are easier to describe and 'respectable'.

Table 14.1 Main features of anxiety and depression

Condition	Main features	
Anxiety	Chief complaints:	all-pervasive apprehension feelings of impending doom panic attacks
	Physical symptoms:	palpitations pain in the chest flushing or pallor difficulty in breathing choking feeling trembling dizziness failure to micturate or defecate
	Psychological symptoms:	irritability fatigue patient easily frustrated hypochondriacal preoccupations
Depression	Severe symptoms:	guilt retardation suicidal feelings
	Useful indications:	loss of interest and enjoyment* poor concentration loss of appetitite* loss of libido* and diurnal variation of mood* loss of weight
	Other factors:	broken sleep or early waking previous episode tiredness—the patient who feels 'tired all the time'

*These factors not typically found together in other psychotic illness.

They therefore tend to conceal their emotions unless directly asked about them. Risk factors relating to suicide are shown in Box 14.2 and indicators of impending suicide in Box 14.3.

Box 14.2 Risk factors related to suicide

- Male sex
- Elderly
- Single
- Widowed or divorced
- Recent bereavement
- Chronic physical illness
- Family history of suicide
- Previous attempts

> **Box 14.3** Indicators of impending suicide
> 1. Life events
> 2. Intractable problems
> 3. Previous attempts
> 4. Premeditation for more than 24 hours
> 5. Patient blames self for his or her predicament
> 6. Patient is manifestly depressed
> 7. Patient complains of severe insomnia
> 8. Patient is losing weight
> 9. Anger
> 10. Social isolation
> 11. Bereavement
> 12. Redundancy
> 13. Abrasive family relationships

A gradual approach is helpful and effective. First, ask how the future seems. Then enquire whether he is worried by thoughts that he might harm himself. Thirdly, say 'Do you feel so bad that you want to harm yourself?' And finally ask him whether he is seriously considering doing away with himself and has he made any specific plans in this regard.

These graded questions allow a fair assessment to be made of the depth of depression. Patients who are truly suicidal do not resent such an approach and answer honestly.

Albert told me that he thought of putting an end to things but has not really got the courage.

Look at the tables again. What were my difficulties?

The first problem was to decide whether he was sufficiently depressed to require urgent admission to hospital. Direct questioning on his intention to commit suicide really did not confirm this. He admitted that his thoughts were only passing ones and were immediately dismissed.

Secondly, how should this man be managed? It was important to show him that I recognized and sympathized with his distress, but that I felt that he had got things out of proportion and that I would try to help him put that right. He needs strong reassurance about his fears of a brain tumour, and this may well come from a thorough examination of his fundi, his

head, neck and reflexes. It was important to reassure him that I would not forget his worries on this score should things not settle down.

The next decision was whether to give him drugs, and this raises the question of the prescription of psychotropes.

The past 20 years have seen the development of powerful antidepressant and anxiolytic drugs. A general practitioner may write 2000 prescriptions for such drugs in one year. There has not however been a parallel clarification of the conditions which respond to them, or clear agreement on the signs and symptoms appropriate to treat. Patients with somatic symptoms like tiredness, early morning waking and weight loss respond best to antidepressants but often the general practitioner is faced with a situation where the best policy is a simple 6 week trial of antidepressant therapy to determine if a given patient will respond. Note that those patients, where anxiety is mixed with depression, respond best to antidepressants rather than tranquillizers.

Drugs used in the treatment of depression

The well-established standard antidepressant was formerly the tricyclic amitriptyline. Unfortunately the tricyclics can have troublesome side-effects (Table 14.3) and newer antidepressants have been developed with different side-effect profiles. General Practitioners would be wise to obtain experience with a handful of the drugs to give sufficient flexibility for patients' requirements. Amitriptyline and dothiepin are sedative and thus useful for patients with sleep problems. Lofepramine is less sedative with fewer anticholinergic side-effects than most tricyclics.

In the last few years antidepressant prescribing has switched to the selective serotonin reuptake inhibitors (SSRIs). These antidepressants have considerable advantages over the tricyclics in that they:

1. are less sedative
2. avoid the anticholinergic side effects of tricyclics
3. are safer in patients who abuse alcohol
4. are free from the cardiotoxicity of tricyclics
5. are safer in overdose.

Nausea is their principle side effect. As a further development we now have the selective noradrenaline reuptake inhibitors (SNRIs). The SSRIs and SNRIs are largely replacing the tricyclics in the treatment of

Table 14.2 SSRIs and SNRIs

Drug	Type	Dose (mg/day)
Citalopram (Cipramil)	SSRI	20–60
Fluoxetine (Prozac)	SSRI	20–60
Fluvoxamine (Faverin)	SSRI	100–300
Mirtazapine (Zispin)	NASSA*	30
Nefazodone (Dutonin)	SSRI	50–600
Paroxetine (Seroxat)	SSRI	20–50
Reboxetine (Edronax)	SNRI	8–12
Sertraline (Lustral)	SSRI	50–200
Venlafaxine (Efexor)	SSRI/SNRI	75–225

*A noradrenaline and selective serotonin antidepressant.

depression. Table 14.2 lists the currently available SRRIs and SNRIs.

In this case I prescribed paroxetine 20 mg/day, warning about the possibility of nausea in the first few days. I arranged to see him again in 10 days and indicated that I was available on the telephone should any difficulties arise. It might also have been prudent to give him the local Samaritan telephone number should he feel desperate in the meantime.

The time scale of likely symptomatic improvement in depression is shown in Figure 14.1. Note that patients should be warned of the slow onset of action of antidepressants (2 weeks) and that any trial of treatment should be for at least 6 weeks.

At the next appointment ask questions to find out the level of his depression, changes in his sleep pattern, bowels, micturition, etc.

When I saw him 2 weeks later he had made a gradual and uneventful recovery. He lost his fears of a brain tumour and has slipped back into his normal daily routine. I learned subsequently that one of the great friends of his youth died of a brain tumour 6 months previously, but he had felt too foolish to mention this to me.

Table 14.3 shows the wide range of side-effects of tricyclic drugs.

This case of mine typifies many of the current dilemmas facing the general practitioner: the problem of the recognition of a new condition in a patient on regular treatment, the assessment of the suicidal risk, the decision to prescribe an antidepressant, the choice of antidepressant, the management and follow-up of the depressed patient, and the decision about the length of treatment necessary. In this context it is as well to remember that 50% of patients with depressive symptoms can relapse spontaneously and that this is cut to 25% by continuing treatment for up to 6 months or longer. The antidepressant should then be withdrawn over 2–3 months.

Attempts to assess the severity of depression have been made, and two useful scales are the *Beck De-*

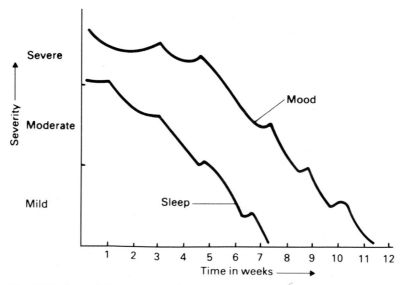

Fig. 14.1 Successful response to antidepressant treatment.

Table 14.3 Side-effects of tricyclic drugs

System	Side-effects
Cardiovascular	Postural hypotension
	Cardiac conductive time lengthened
	Quinidine-like effect—a/v block
	Arrhythmias
	Tachycardia
CNS	Drowsiness: lessens after 1–2 weeks
	Confusion—atropine-like
	Fine tremor, especially in the elderly
	Lower convulsive threshold
	Pupils dilate
	Raised intra-ocular pressure
	Hyperhidrosis, especially imipramine
Metabolic	Weight gain
	Lower blood glucose
	Menstrual irregularities
	Jaundice
Gastrointestinal	Constipation
	Reduced stomach acid secretion
	(dyspepsia can improve)
Genitourinary	Urinary retention
	Delayed orgasm

pression Inventory and the *Hamilton Rating Scale.* These are readily available and are included here as Appendices A and B. Reading through the Beck Depression Inventory is an excellent way to remind oneself how a patient experiences depression.

TEACHING POINTS

1. Patients under regular care can become depressed.
2. The assessment of suicidal risk is important.
3. The decision to prescribe antidepressants depends on the assessment of risk and the severity of the depression.
4. The management and follow-up of a depressed patient is crucial.
5. The decision to treat depends on many factors.

15 DIARRHOEA

Diarrhoea may be defined as a deviation from the established bowel rhythm characterized by an increase in the frequency and fluidity of the stools.

The significance of this definition will be appreciated when it is remembered that 99% of people defecate between three times a day and once in 3 days. In the population, 3% may have had diarrhoea within the previous fortnight, and in a London borough 7% had diarrhoea at the time of the survey. One in four patients treated the condition themselves and one in seven consulted their doctors. Diarrhoea is the fifth most common presenting symptom in general practice and an average general practitioner may expect to see 125 cases a year.

In 1998 considerable media interest was shown in the outbreaks of *Escherichia coli* 0157 infection in Scotland; 501 people were affected, of whom 20 died. Concern is justified because the incidence of food poisoning is continuing to rise. The figures have risen continuously since 1980. The number of laboratory reports of campylobacter and salmonella isolated has risen threefold since that time.

E. coli may appear in two forms: Vero cytotoxin *E. coli* (VTEC positive) and *E. coli* without Vero cytotoxin (non-VTEC). *E. coli* (VTEC) has typical symptoms of diarrhoea, vomiting, abdominal pain, bloody diarrhoea/urine, kidney failure; it is carried in uncooked meat, raw milk and cheese, and the usual incubation period is 24–36 hours. Non-VTEC *E. coli* usually presents as diarrhoea only and is found in salad, raw milk, vegetables and cheese and has a 24–48-hour incubation period.

Mrs Crooks brought in her 5-year-old daughter Susan with diarrhoea.

What questions would you ask?

1. How long has she had it?
2. How many bowel motions a day?
3. The consistency of the stool?
4. Is there any blood?
5. Accompanied by vomiting?
6. Any contact with other cases of diarrhoea?
7. Are the rest of the family well?

The purpose of these questions is to identify diarrhoea of recent onset and to assess its severity. An important clue is the presence or absence of blood, and questions about vomiting are helpful in gauging the likelihood of dehydration.

What is an appropriate examination?

As the patient often requests advice about diarrhoea on the telephone it is important to be clear in our own minds what we are seeking. Diarrhoea is a common condition and many cases present themselves to a doctor, the majority being mild self-limiting conditions due to common causes (Box 15.1). Dietary indiscretion or a mild virus infection are the most likely. In these conditions the doctor's task is to be alert to the more serious conditions which either present as diarrhoea or may develop from it—for example, acute appendicitis or dehydration. At an early stage the doctor should seek to identify clues which single out the more serious problems and be prepared to follow them closely, while expecting the majority to settle with minimal supervision. In one practice, 5.2% of the population had diarrhoea and 84% were examined bacteriologically. Sonne dysentery was found in 0.4%, except during an outbreak when it rose to 29%.

What examination would you make?

The appearance of the patient creates a strong and important impression on the examining doctor. In a very young or very old patient or one who looks ill or debilitated, the doctor is much more likely to seek other causes. In a fit, healthy-looking adult with no apparent dehydration it is unlikely that even a cursory

Box 15.1   Causes of acute diarrhoea

- *Infections*
  Gastrointestinal
  Viral: Echovirus
              Coxsackie
              Rotavirus
              Others
  Bacterial: Cholera
              Dysentery—*Shigella sonne*
              Salmonella: typhoid
                          paratyphoid
              Campylobacter
              Escherichia coli
              Endotoxin—staphylococcal
              food poisoning
              Exotoxin—clostridial food
              poisoning
  Protozoal: *Giardia lamblia*
              Entamoeba histolytica
  Other infections   Upper respiratory tract
                     infections
                     Acute appendicitis

- *Dietary indiscretion*
              Unripe fruit
              Alcohol excess
              Unaccustomed holiday diet
              Artificial feeding in babies
  Escherichia coli
              Endotoxin—Staphylococcal
              food poisoning
              Exotoxin—Clostridial food
              poisoning

- *Allergy*

- *Diverticulitis*

- *Psychological*

- *Drugs*   Antibiotics
              Magnesium trisilicate
              Laxatives
              Hypotensives

abdominal palpation will be indicated. However, in omitting this examination the doctor should be aware that he or she is consciously not seeking confirmatory

abdominal tenderness or a mass. This habit of deliberately discarding an opportunity to obtain a piece of confirmatory evidence should sharpen your thoughts about the working diagnosis you have made. In Susan's case, as she is a child, it is wise to palpate the abdomen. Having done this you decide that this is probably a mild self-limiting infective condition which will resolve spontaneously. If it does not settle within 24–48 hours you must review the diagnosis and be aware that acute appendicitis can progress too far in this time. The mother must understand under what circumstances a further request for medical advice should be made. In essence you are distinguishing between diarrhoea of recent onset (i.e. with a history of 24–48 hours only) and other presentations.

Investigation

It might be argued that with so much doubt in each case a bacteriological examination of the stool should be made, but consider the arguments:

1. The number of positive results in the examination of the stool is of the order of 9%.
2. The number of carriers in the community is unknown and therefore the value of a positive result is difficult to assess.
3. The problem of collecting and transferring large quantities of potentially infectious material.
4. The average cost of each laboratory test.

All this has to be equated with the assistance given to the doctor in making a clinical decision. A rational approach would be to investigate those cases which are suspect, either because there is blood in the stool or because the patient has a job in the food industry or has made a recent visit abroad. Other possibilities might be the inmates of various institutions because of the risk to a closed community, the immunosuppressed and those in whom food poisoning is suspected.

Management

In the management of diarrhoea, especially in children, it is important to reassure the parents that this is likely to be a self-limiting condition and not due to a serious cause.

The three main points to consider are:

1. dehydration

Table 15.1   Electrolyte and sugar solutions

Solution	Flavours
Dioralyte	Plain, citrus or blackcurrant
Electrolade	Banana, melon, orange or blackcurrant
Rehidrat	Orange, blackcurrant or lemon/lime

2. diet
3. drugs.

Dehydration. The safest and simplest way to replace fluid loss is with an electrolyte and sugar solution, of which there are several available in sachet form (Table 15.1).

Diet. Food can be allowed as soon as the appetite permits. The special solution will supply all the nourishment needed as it contains glucose. If vomiting is a problem, reduction in the quantity and increase in the frequency of administration of the solution will often overcome this. Stress the importance of a high fluid intake. Parents should be told that persistent vomiting for longer than 24 hours should be reported to you.

Drugs. These play little part in the treatment of diarrhoea and should be avoided altogether in children. In adults antimotility drugs such as loperamide (Imodium) may be used for symptomatic treatment of diarrhoea. Antibiotics are of no use except in the following rare situations:

1. Acute traveller's diarrhoea, when ciprofloxacin may be helpful.
2. Campylobacter infection, where erythromycin 500 mg q.d.s. for 7 days can be prescribed.
3. *Giardia lamblia* infection where metronidazole 2 g daily for 3 days, repeated in 14 days, is the treatment.
4. Severe salmonella, shigella or *E. coli* infection.
5. For the treatment of *Clostridium difficile*.

RECURRENT DIARRHOEA

The management of recurrent diarrhoea is quite different. Box 15.2 is an aide-memoire for the likely causes.

Box 15.2   Chronic diarrhoea

An illness of more than 1–2 weeks' duration. The probabilities are dependent on the age of the patient

1. Old age	Superior mesenteric artery thrombosis
2. Late middle age	Neoplasm, diverticulitis
3. Young adult	Ulcerative colitis, Crohn's disease, metabolic disease such as diabetes, Addison's disease or thyrotoxicosis
4. Children	Coeliac disease
5. In anyone	Iatrogenic diarrhoea, bowel surgery, chronic anxiety

For Susan I prescribed bed rest, plenty of fluids, no solid foods, no school, with a gradual return to normal in 3 or 4 days. Mrs Crooks returned in 2 days' time to say that her daughter had a cough.

This is a frequent turn of events and probably indicates that the girl is suffering from a respiratory virus. Provided the diarrhoea has stopped and there is no other indication of illness, symptomatic treatment would be appropriate.

However, at this juncture, Mrs Crooks mentions that her daughter has lost weight.

What would you do next?

Further history should indicate why she has made this remark, whether it is a recent or longstanding problem and whether there have been any upsets in the family. At this consultation it would be sensible to weigh Susan, enquire about home, school, diet, etc., and make a further appointment to weigh her again in 3–4 weeks. It would also help to check her growth against a percentile chart, as a low reading would be a clue to a chronic condition. It should also be noted that this series of consultations has changed in its form.

The girl presented with a symptom, diarrhoea, developed another, a cough, and the mother then shows anxiety over her weight. Is the real reason for the consultations the mother's fears about her child's development, and would this be a more fruitful area of enquiry? The importance of a management plan against which changes can be measured can now be appreciated.

INFANTILE GASTROENTERITIS

Diarrhoea in infants is a common cause of consultation. It may, however, be serious and babies can become severely dehydrated quickly with serious consequences, including fitting. It is thus essential to recognize signs of dehydration in a baby. This is best done by weighing the child at the onset; a subsequent loss of weight indicates significant and severe dehydration. The main principle is one of suitable fluid with nothing else by mouth.

History

What is the mother using to replace the fluids lost through diarrhoea and vomiting? If replacing with solids and milk, suspect hypernatraemic dehydration.

Examination

Exclude other infections, especially meningitis. Excess vomiting is suspicious. Remember intussusception.

Approach

When faced with this problem the management plan given in Figure 15.1 is useful as a guide.

TEACHING POINTS
1. Distinguish between acute, subacute and chronic diarrhoea.
2. Know the causes of diarrhoea.
3. Practical points for action:
   a. blood in the stool,
   b. the presence of illness,
   c. weight loss,
   d. history of contact.
4. Always look for signs of dehydration in infants.

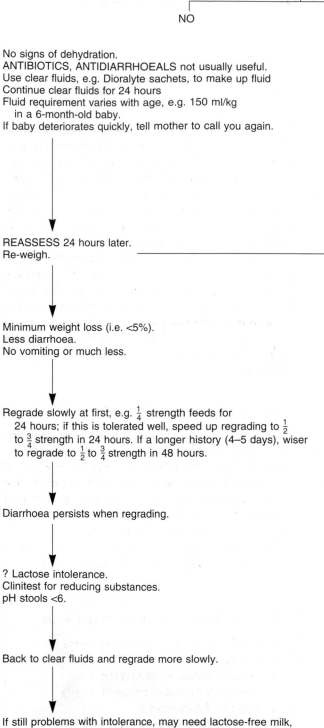

DOES THE BABY LOOK ILL?

NO

YES

No signs of dehydration.
ANTIBIOTICS, ANTIDIARRHOEALS not usually useful.
Use clear fluids, e.g. Dioralyte sachets, to make up fluid
Continue clear fluids for 24 hours
Fluid requirement varies with age, e.g. 150 ml/kg
    in a 6-month-old baby.
If baby deteriorates quickly, tell mother to call you again.

(i) Signs of dehydration e.g., sunken eyes, sunken
    fontanelle, obvious weight loss, doughy skin
                        OR
(ii) Drowsy baby
                        OR
(iii) Other suspected illness.

HOSPITAL

REASSESS 24 hours later.
Re-weigh.

Weight loss substantial in 24 hours (i.e. >5%).
Symptoms unabated or worse.
Signs of dehydration.

Minimum weight loss (i.e. <5%).
Less diarrhoea.
No vomiting or much less.

Regrade slowly at first, e.g. $\frac{1}{4}$ strength feeds for
    24 hours; if this is tolerated well, speed up regrading to $\frac{1}{2}$
    to $\frac{3}{4}$ strength in 24 hours. If a longer history (4–5 days), wiser
    to regrade to $\frac{1}{2}$ to $\frac{3}{4}$ strength in 48 hours.

Diarrhoea persists when regrading.

? Lactose intolerance.
Clinitest for reducing substances.
pH stools <6.

Back to clear fluids and regrade more slowly.

If still problems with intolerance, may need lactose-free milk,
    and may need referral.

Fig. 15.1 Management plan for diarrhoea in a baby

16 SKIN INFECTIONS AND INFESTATIONS

Most doctors will be familiar with the presentation and treatment of the major skin diseases, eczema and psoriasis, and will experience little difficulty in managing boils, cellulitis and impetigo. This leaves a mixed bag of minor conditions treated less well and which are less familiar to the young doctor. Acne and warts are dealt with in Chapter 3, and here we deal with fungal infections. Fungal skin infections are seen regularly in general practice. They can be severe and extensive in immunologically compromised patients, and the increase in bone marrow transplantation and AIDS means that general practitioners are increasingly likely to see more severe examples.

Ringworm is in fact a loose term for a group of fungus infections, but it is a term the public understand and the patient often suspects the diagnosis. The more precise medical terminology relates the infection to the part of the body affected; hence tinea pedis, tinea cruris, etc.

Finally we look at some common infections/infestations seen in practice. All the conditions mentioned in this chapter can be diagnosed without a microscope, but this aid certainly makes practice more fun if you have one!

James Torcross, a 24-year-old bank clerk, keen on squash and rugby, came to the surgery one afternoon complaining of an irritating rash in his groin. It had been present for 2 weeks and he had been told by a relation who was a nurse that it was probably ringworm and that he ought to come to the surgery for treatment. On examination there was a small circular red patch on the left upper thigh adjacent to the scrotum; it was quite scaly with a densely red raised edge, although centrally it was pinker with fewer scales.

What are the possible diagnoses?

The differential diagnosis seems to lie between intertrigo, psoriasis and tinea cruris (ringworm). Psoriasis looks different from the classical annular shape of ringworm and there may be other lesions elsewhere. Intertrigo is usually found in the inguinal fold, not on the thigh, and often has associated weeping. In established lesions ringworm is usually readily recognized; particularly note the raised red scaly edge and the history of outward spread of the lesion. If at all in doubt the diagnosis can be confirmed by examination of some skin scrapings taken from near the edge of the lesion and placed on a slide with 10% potassium hydroxide; after soaking for a few minutes the fungal hyphae will be easily seen on microscopic examination. Ringworm of the groin (*tinea cruris*) is usually caused by one of three species of fungus—*Trichophyton rubrum*, *Trichophyton interdigitale* or *Epidermophyton floccosum*.

Is there any further examination desirable?

Tinea cruris is often associated with tinea pedis—the same fungi can cause both and infection can spread from the feet; often both are present together. If foot ringworm were better controlled it is likely that the incidence of tinea cruris would also fall. It is thus reasonable to examine the feet. If the diagnosis is in doubt examine other areas of the skin.

There is a wide differential diagnosis for erythematous annular lesions on the skin (Box 16.1).

Box 16.1 Annular erythematous eruptions on the skin

- Dermatophyte infections (ringworm)
- Annular urticaria (not scaly)
- Subacute lupus erythematosus (rare)
- Granuloma annulare (not scaly)
- Annular lichen planus
- Erythema chronicum migrans (in Lyme disease—extremely rare)

Mr Torcross was curious about his illness and asked the following questions. How would you respond?

Is it very infectious?

Tinea cruris can be caught from infected clothes and the fungus is difficult to eradicate from underclothes. The sharing of bathing trunks, sports clothes, etc., is one way in which infection can spread and it is worth pointing this out to a young athletic patient. In the normal course of events it is probably not very infectious and it is relatively rare to see more than one member of the family affected. It is probably worthwhile advising use of separate towels and boiling of infected clothes separately from the rest of the family's clothes.

I have a dog at home—could I have caught it from him?

Ringworm fungi can be divided into geophilic (originating in the soil), zoophilic (with animal origins) and anthropophilic species (largely confined to humans). All the fungi causing *tinea cruris* tend to be anthropophilic: it is thus unlikely to be contracted from a dog. However, in some forms of ringworm, infection may originate from animals.

Will it affect my genitals?

Scrotal involvement is relatively common and occasionally it can involve the penis. Treatment will prevent this.

How would you treat a case like this?

The growth of ringworm is encouraged by sweating and friction from clothes, which may themselves be infected. Clean loose-fitting undergarments should be worn, with every attempt made to reduce perspiration in the area. It is also sensible to boil any clothing directly in contact with the lesion, i.e. underpants and pyjamas.

Small localized patches of tinea cruris respond well to topical antifungal preparations such as miconazole (Daktarin), econazole (Ecostatin), clotrimazole (Canesten) or terbinafine (Lamisil) cream. With severe surrounding inflammation use the preparations containing antifungal and 1% hydrocortisone cream (e.g. Daktacort).

Any chronic fair-sized lesion will probably need oral therapy. Griseofulvin used to be the established therapy but there are now quicker-acting agents available with fewer side-effects. An example of the newer agents is oral terbinafine therapy which requires:

- one tablet daily for 2–6 weeks for tinea pedis
- one tablet daily for 2–4 weeks for tinea cruris
- one tablet daily for 4 weeks for tinea corporis
- one tablet daily for 6–12 weeks for fingernail infections
- one tablet daily for 3–6 months for toenail infections.

See the literature for contraindications and drug interactions.

Unfortunately tinea cruris does tend to relapse, largely due to the persistence of a hot, sweaty environment and friction from tight clothes; patients should be warned of this. It is interesting to note that if steroid creams are mistakenly used as the sole treatment the lesion will spread rapidly (and atypically), emphasizing once more the good principles of examination, diagnosis, investigation and appropriate treatment.

Peter Skelson had an irritating peeling of the skin between his toes; he guessed it had been there 3 months. He thought it was a 'sweat rash' and wanted some ointment to put on it.

On examination of his feet you find white peeling and macerated skin between the toe clefts, more marked on one foot than the other, being largely confined to three lateral toe clefts on the right foot. What are the possible diagnoses?

Tinea pedis (foot ringworm, 'athlete's foot') commonly presents in this way as a maceration, scaling and fissuring on the webs of the little toes (rarely between the first and second toe). It is the commonest fungal infection of the skin and is particularly prevalent in young adult males. There are three species commonly responsible: *Trichophyton rubrum*, *Trichophyton interdigitale* and *Epidermophyton floccosum*. Depending on the species and the degree of secondary bacterial infection, it is possible for it to present as a wide variety of eruptions on the toes or on the whole of the foot, including the sole. There are in particular severe blistering forms, hyperkeratotic forms and pustular forms. The nails may also be affected but usually the dorsum of the foot is spared.

In a young child, infected eczema of the toes is a possibility, but this has a different distribution, usually extending to the dorsum of the foot, whereas the peeling of ringworm tends to extend to the plantar surface.

Similar changes to ringworm, particularly in the toe cleft area, can be produced by other organisms, including *Corynebacterium minutissimum* (erythasma) and candidiasis.

The combination of a sweaty foot and ill-fitting shoes can also produce macerated scaling. The picture here is more symmetrical, often involves the dorsum of the toes and is largely confined to the space between the surfaces of the fourth and fifth toes. If in doubt the scales can be examined for fungus, as described.

Are there any predisposing factors to foot ringworm and is it very infectious?

Excessive sweating of the feet and tight-fitting shoes will provide a good environment for fungal growth. The fungus can be transmitted by infected scales of skin and hence is more common in certain groups of people, e.g. those in institutions and those using communal bathing facilities and changing rooms. Especially prone will be miners, athletes, students in schools and universities. The swimming bath is another potential source of infection. There must be some host resistance, as among families, using the same bathroom, cross-infection is not very common.

How would you treat tinea pedis?

The varied manifestations of foot ringworm mean that the approach to treatment has to fit the problem. An acute severe inflammation of the feet with vesicles and exudate may best initially be treated with potassium permanganate (1:8000) soaks for 10 minutes every 4 hours.

The more common toe-web infection, as in this case, can be very resistant to treatment and the relapse rate is high, especially in hot weather. Miconazole cream can be applied in the web spaces, with oral or topical terbinafine a useful alternative, although relapses may occur when therapy is discontinued.

As well as this therapy it is wise to educate the patient to prevent relapses as far as possible. Suitable advice would include the following:

1. Buy new woollen socks and change frequently.

2. Wash and dry feet well at least once a day. Mopping with surgical spirit and dusting with talcum powder has been recommended by some.
3. Use sensible footwear, preferably of the 'open' type.
4. Use slippers rather than walk barefoot on any communal floor to prevent reinfection.

On a community basis, frequent washing of changing room floors, use of antifungal powders at swimming pools, etc., would help, but the ubiquitous nature of the fungus makes it difficult. Patients continue to return for their regular prescription for ointment despite all measures taken.

We have seen ringworm of the groin and foot. Where else can ringworm be found?

1. Hands: rare.
2. Nails (tinea unguium): distinguish from psoriasis and the chronic phronychia of *Candida albicans*. Over 2% of the adult population is thought to have some fungal nail infestation. The estimated cost of eradicating this is £500 million. There are effective synthetic antifungals with cure rates of more than 80%. Long-term antifungal treatment should not be used as a diagnostic tool. The rational approach seems to be sure of the diagnosis, be cost effective and use the new and powerful drugs carefully. Demonstration of fungus in nail clippings by microscopy is sufficient evidence to start treatment. Choice of treatment depends on the patient's age/preference/number of nails affected/degree of involvement and other drugs being taken.
3. Body (tinea corporis): look for the typical ringed lesions. Can be caught from cattle (cattle ringworm in farmers).
4. Scalp (tinea capitis): mainly children. Woods light demonstrates. Contagious in schools when passed from child to child but can also be caught from cats or dogs.
5. Beard (tinea barbae).

INFESTATIONS

Below are three consultations. In each case, identify the most likely parasite responsible and describe the symptoms caused, the means of diagnosis and the management. The answers are in Table 16.1.

Case 1. A mother brings her young child to you in the surgery saying that he has been scratching himself around the anal region at night and she thinks he has worms.

Case 2. A mother has brought her child to you complaining that he is continually scratching his scalp. On examination you see a few white flecks on the hairs looking like dandruff.

Case 3. A 40-year-old patient comes to your surgery complaining of severe generalized itching, worse on going to bed. On examination you find a red papular rash on the trunk and around the axillae. There are also excoriated scaly lesions between the fingers.

TEACHING POINTS

1. Ringworm is usually a 'spot' diagnosis but can be confirmed by examining skin scrapings on a microscope slide with 10% potassium hydroxide.
2. Learn how to prescribe antifungal agents.
3. Tinea pedis can present as a wide variety of lesions and eruptions on the foot and toes but usually the dorsum is spared.
4. Relapses of tinea pedis are common and all patients should be advised on simple measures they can adopt.
5. Threadworms are common and usually present as pruritus ani in a young child.
6. If head lice are found, inform the Health Visitor.
7. Remember scabies as a cause of pruritus.
8. A miscroscope in your practice can be useful.

Table 16.1   Three common infestations

	Incidence and aetiology	Symptoms	Diagnosis	Management
Threadworms (*Enterobius vermicularis*)	Commonest worm infestation. About 40% of children below 10	1. Mostly asymptomatic 2. Pruritus ani as eggs laid by gravid females at night on perianal skin 3. Worms passed in stool 4. Vulvovaginitis 5. Insomnia and irritability, secondary to (2)	1. Worms in stool 2. Child attends morning surgery with no prior washing of skin. Sellotape (sticky side out) on a tongue depressor pressed on perianal skin then tape transferred to microscope slide	1. Treat all the family 2. Hygiene. Keep nails short and scrubbed clean. Bathe thoroughly. Clean toilet thoroughly. Regular changing of underclothing and bed linen 3. Drugs; treat family. Either Pripsen: over 6 years one sachet (10 g), 1–6 years ⅔ sachet, 3 months– 1 year ⅓ sachet. Single dose repeated after 14 days; or mebendazole (Vermox): 1 tablet of 100 mg or suspension of 100 mg repeated in 2–3 weeks. Not for under 2 years old
Head lice (*Pediculus capitis*)	Often found on school inspection as eggs (nits) in the hair. Louse lives on scalp. Spread by close contact	1. Scalp irritation (often secondary infection due to the scratching) 2. Asymptomatic	1. Can sometimes see lice 2. Eggs or nits; small white specks attached to hair shaft. Unlike dandruff can't be brushed off. Examination with microscope confirms hair	Malathion 0.5% (Prioderm, Derbac), phenothrin (Full Marks) or permethrin (Lyclear) are treatment options. Apply Prioderm lotion to hair, rub in and leave to dry. Twelve hours later shampoo and comb with a fine -toothed metal comb. Repeat after one week. Inform Health Visitor and Community Medical Officer so others in the school can be treated

Table 16.1   Three common infestations (continued)

	Incidence and aetiology	Symptoms	Diagnosis	Management
Scabies (Sarcoptes scabei)	Infection of skin with a mite, Sarcoptes scabei, burrowing into epidermis. Transferred by close bodily contact, hence often a family history. In the elderly or in institutions Norwegian scabies may be found (presents as a general red scaling)	Initially may be none, but after 4 weeks generalized irritation worse at night. Subsequently a red papular rash which may be generalized. Scratching may lead to secondary eczematous changes and secondary bacterial infection is common	Look for the burrows with hand lens; usually 0.5 cm grey linear scaly lesion. May also present as papular urticarial eruption. Sites for burrows are between the fingers, anterior aspect of wrists, axillary folds, borders of the palms. Rare on face or scalp. Take scrapings with blunt scalpel to look under microscope for mites and eggs	1. Treat family and all contacts 2. Benzylbenzoate BP or permethrin for adults but permethrin (Lyclear dermal cream) for children, as benzylbenzoate is irritant. See manufacturer's leaflet for precise instructions on use 3. Note that itching may continue long after scabies has been cured

The Health Visitor is useful in checking out and advising families.
The absence of a microscope need not handicap efficient diagnosis in the presence of typical histories and signs.

17 THE RED EYE

A patient presenting with a red eye is always worrying as the diagnosis may be a serious one with a risk of permanent blindness. However, the majority of conditions are relatively minor and easily managed. Patients, on the other hand, may have their own ideas about the significance of the condition, and if this is not recognized, it will make successful management very difficult. Patients with eye diseases constitute 8% of all consultations. The average general practitioner may expect to see 110 people with eye disease each year. Between 5 and 10% of all attendances at Accident and Emergency Departments are for ophthalmic problems. There is seasonal variation, and conjunctivitis may occur in epidemics.

George Cropston, a dapper, middle-aged gentleman, consults you one morning saying: 'I've come about my eye, doctor. It's gone red.'

What do you do next?

A rapid glance confirmed that he had indeed an inflamed eye.

What questions should you ask?

The history

If you take a careful history the patient will tell you when and how the eye became red. Important questions are:

- How long have you had it?
- Is it getting worse?
- Have you had anything like this before?
- Do you suffer from any allergies or hay fever?
- Is there a discharge? If so, is it watery, or does it contain pus?
- Is there any itching?
- Have you got any pain?
- Has there been any disturbance of vision?

- Are there any other symptoms, or is there a constitutional upset?
- Have you had any vomiting?
- Is there any possibility that you have something in it?
- Were you hammering or chiselling at the time (metallic foreign bodies being important to exclude)?

In the examination, what specific observations should you make?

The examination

Always start with a general examination of the patient. Does he look worried, ill or pale? Could there be a systemic illness?

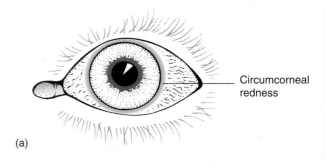

(a)

Circumcorneal redness

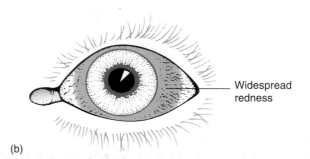

(b)

Widespread redness

Fig. 17.1 A Circumcorneal redness; **B** Widespread redness.

Now turn to the eye. Compare it with the other eye. This will show whether the condition is bilateral; if it is not, it also indicates what might be considered as normal anatomy. A general inspection will show where the redness is (Fig. 17.1). Is it around the margin of the iris or is the whole conjunctiva affected? This is a key observation in the decision to refer. Is the eye hard? Palpate it.

Now examine the pupil. Is it regular or irregular? Does it respond to light? Check the depth of the anterior chamber by the eclipse test (Fig. 17.2). Check the central vision with a pin-hole disc (Fig. 17.3). Check the field of vision with simple hand movements (Fig. 17.4) in the surrounding fields.

The lids—are they inflamed? What is under the eyelid? Evert the upper eyelid by taking the lashes

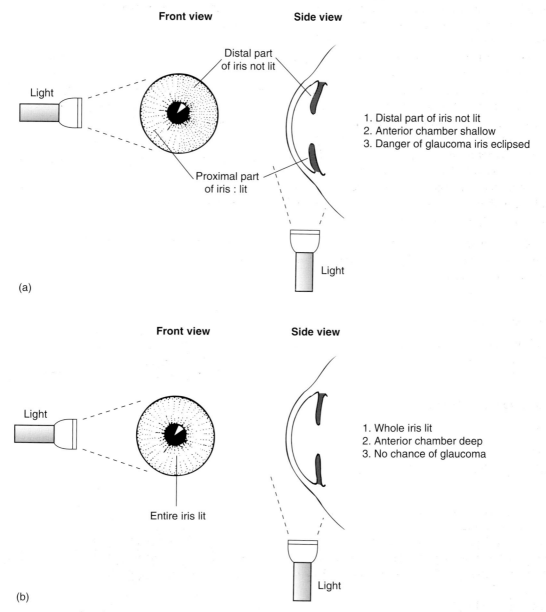

Fig. 17.2 The eclipse test. **A** Anterior chamber shallow; iris 'eclipsed'; danger of glaucoma. **B** Entire iris lit. Anterior chamber deep; iris lit; no glaucoma.

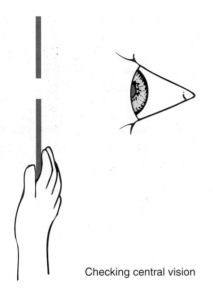

Checking central vision

Fig. 17.3 Checking central vision.

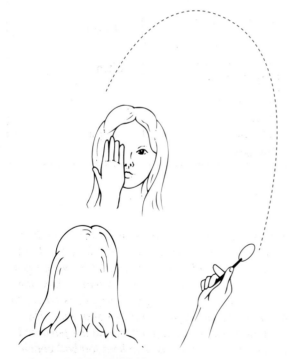

Fig. 17.4 Checking visual field.

in your fingers and everting over a glass rod or similar object. Look for discharge: is it purulent?

Is the cornea affected? Circumcorneal redness is the hallmark of serious red eye problems (see below,

Treat or refer?). Is the corneal epithelium intact? Cornea without epithelium stains; intact epithelium does not (see below, the use of fluorescein).

Complete the examination with one drop of Minims Fluorescein and examine with a torch. Take care with patients who wear contact lenses (these can be damaged by taking up the fluorescein stain). An abrasion with or without a foreign body will be seen. Herpetic ulcers will stain with a typical dendritic pattern.

Differential diagnosis

The problem is to distinguish an allergic or infective conjunctivitis starting in one eye, from serious conditions such as iritis, glaucoma and keratitis. The main points to bear in mind are that conjunctivitis is usually bilateral, associated with discharge and/or itching; the pupil is normal and vision is unaffected. The diagnostic features of these conditions are shown in Table 17.1.

Redness and discharge

It is important to recognize that the degree, depth and extent of the redness is no guide to the severity of the underlying condition. True infective conjunctivitis is usually bilateral and the presence of discharge is a very helpful diagnostic point. It may be minimal and be represented only by stickiness of the lids, or it can be profuse and last for between 1 and 6 days. A purulent discharge from one eye alone really represents a different scale of urgency.

Visual acuity

A recent change in visual acuity is the best guide to the urgency of the situation.

All doctors should possess the means of testing vision with an appropriate Snellen's chart. The test chart should be viewed from a distance of 6 metres (20 feet), or 3 metres (10 feet) if a mirror is used. The last line the patient can read is the visual acuity for that eye. Each row is calibrated against the distance at which it can be read by the normal eye; these are the figures which appear on the charts. Thus if only the top line can be read at 6 metres the visual acuity would be 6:60; normal visual acuity would be 6:6.

The recorded loss of one line of the standard chart is significant if it occurs within a short period of time.

Table 17.1   The differential diagnosis of a red eye

	Acute conjunctivitis	Acute iritis	Acute glaucoma	Keratitis
Pain	Gritty	Yes, boring	Severe	Yes
Discharge	Yes; can be profuse	Reflex watering	Reflex watering	Yes
Visual disturbance	Smeared with discharge	Yes	Gross	Yes
Visual acuity	Normal	Reduced, blurred	Reduced	Normal or reduced
Site of inflammation	Peripheral	Circumcorneal	Diffuse purplish	Diffuse or circumcorneal
Pupil shape	Normal	Constricted, irregular poor reflex	Dilated, oval, fixed	Normal
Cornea	Clear	Hazy	Steamy	Ulcer
Photophobia	No	Yes	Yes	
Intraocular pressure	Normal	Normal	Raised, eye hard	Normal
Number of patients seen by an average general practitioner in 1 year	45	3	3	3

Pain

The combination of visual disturbance and pain is significant and indicates a serious and urgent presentation. Always look for an ingrowing eyelash. A painful white eye is a sign of a neurological condition, e.g. multiple sclerosis. The differential diagnosis of a painful eye includes conjunctivitis (gritty sensation rather than pain), iritis and glaucoma.

Foreign body

The possibility of a foreign body must always be considered and its detection may be greatly simplified if fluorescein drops are used (see above). It is important to ask concerning a history of hammering or chiselling metallic objects or other possible sources of foreign bodies.

Terminology

The nomenclature of various eye conditions is confusing. Figure 17.5 shows the anatomical structures in the eye and their relationship to each other. The uveal tract comprises the iris, the ciliary body, the ciliary muscle and the choroid. Special equipment is required to examine it.

Anterior uveitis = iritis or choroiditis
Posterior uveitis = choroiditis

Box 17.1 summarizes the threat to sight of various conditions.

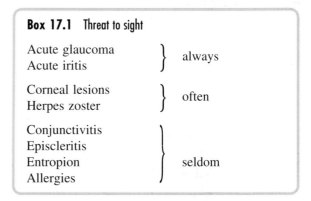

Box 17.1   Threat to sight

Acute glaucoma Acute iritis	} always
Corneal lesions Herpes zoster	} often
Conjunctivitis Episcleritis Entropion Allergies	} seldom

Further questioning reveals that Mr Cropston is a shopkeeper. He has pain in his eye, there has been no discharge, but he has noticed that his vision is a little blurred. Examination reveals that he has some photophobia, the iris is slightly hazy, he is tender to palpation and the pupil is a little constricted. He says that he has had conjunctivitis in the past, and his notes show that he used to be a football coach. He had an episode of low back pain 10 years ago when he was referred to the orthopaedic department. His ESR was 2 mm at that stage and a lumbosacral spine X-ray was normal. However, he did have a raised serum uric acid.

Three months ago he saw one of your partners and a diagnosis of acute conjunctivitis was made.

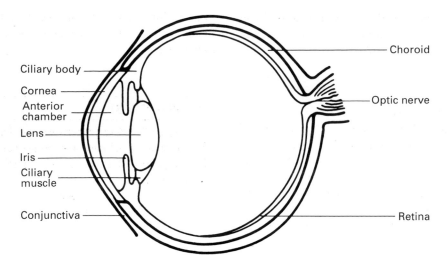

Fig. 17.5 The main structures of the eye. Note: the uveal tract comprises the iris, ciliary body, ciliary muscle and choroid. Anterior uveitis = iritis or iridocyclitis; posterior uveitis = choroiditis

What is your opinion?

In view of the lack of discharge, the fact that he has blurred vision, and that there is unilateral injection around the iris, you consider a provisional diagnosis of iritis. You then refer him urgently for a specialist opinion.

The letter you receive some 2 weeks later indicates that he indeed has uveitis. A blood test shows that the human lymphocyte antigen B27 is present. An X-ray of his lumbosacral spine suggests ankylosing spondylitis. He was treated with steroid eye drops and atropine.

Table 17.2 When to refer red eye conditions to hospital

	If suspected	If diagnosed	Prereferral diagnosis	Only if fails to respond	Atypical features making diagnosis difficult and referral necessary
Dacryoadenitis				+	
Warts					+
Styes (hordeolum)				+	
Chalazion				Rarely	
Blepharitis			Swab and sensitivities		Very persistent
Conjunctivitis				+	Other disease suspected
Acute iritis	+	+			
Acute glaucoma	+	+E T pilocarpine 4%			
Keratitis	+	+			
Foreign body	+	+			Not visible
Corneal ulcer	+	+			
Uveitis	+	+			

+, Referral; E, emergency; T, emergency treatment

In the management of the red eye it is useful to know the indications for specialist referral and these are summarized in Table 17.2.

Treat or refer?

Widespread redness means treatment in primary care is usually possible. The limbal vessels may be red but this feature will not dominate. The most common causes are conjunctivitis, blepharitis, subconjunctival haemorrhage or dry eye syndrome.

Circumcorneal redness is the hallmark of serious eye disease. These vessels are swollen from blood inside the eye. Limbal inflammation means one of three serious causes of the red eye: keratitis, iritis (anterior uveitis) or glaucoma. All need to be referred to hospital.

TEACHING POINTS

1. Learn to differentiate between the causes of a red eye.
2. Pain, discharge and visual acuity are key pointers.
3. Acute glaucoma, keratitis, foreign bodies and corneal ulceration require special care.
4. Conjunctivitis is usually bilateral.
5. Learn appropriate eye preparations.

18 BACKACHE

Acute back pain is another of the common symptoms presented in family practice. An average practitioner might see two new cases a week. Although some statistics estimate 50 new consultations a year for an average practice, this is probably an underestimate. Comfort can be gained from the certain fact that in the great majority—well over three-quarters—symptoms disappear within 4 weeks with analgesia alone and much less than 1 in a 100 attacks requires surgery. Backache is a potent cause of loss of work and the problem of sickness certification arises with this symptom more than with most. It is a symptom which almost more than any other causes a doctor's morale to sink, and recurrent back pain even more. To the patient, backache is sometimes a nuisance, sometimes disabling and occasionally an intolerable burden. It is a reflection of our relative therapeutic impotence that some patients in the end seek the advice of the various paramedical disciplines.

Elsie Liberty was in her 40 s. She worked as a canteen assistant and was a patient familiar to the practice. She had been troubled by back pain once before, but this had responded to simple analgesics and her back had not been the subject of a consultation for many years. Now she hobbled painfully into the consulting room, literally supported by her husband. She was clearly in pain. She complained of severe low back pain and shooting pains down the legs, especially the left one: 'It feels as though my back is on fire,' she groaned. She had twinges of pain the previous day but now the pain had grown in severity so that she could hardly stand. She could not remember exactly how it started, but there was no history of injury. She removed several layers of clothes with difficulty so that I could examine her. She had a slightly tilted spine and was tender over most of the lower back. She could not perform any spinal movements and I did not pursue the matter. I persuaded her with her husband's help to lie on the couch. I found straight leg raising grossly reduced to about 30° on the left, but it was surprisingly good on the right. She was in such pain that she could barely lie still on the couch. The examination of the reflexes was difficult, but I attempted it and thought both knee and ankle reflexes were present. I diagnosed a possible lumbar disc prolapse and explained to her that she had probably a slipped disc.

What are the more common causes of low back pain and what features would you look for in the history in diagnosing a prolapsed intervertebral disc as a cause of backache?

Table 18.1 sets out simply the more common causes of low back pain. The largest group is the one with minor 'musculoskeletal' problems labelled variously as 'fibrositis', 'muscular strain', 'ligament strain', etc. It will be obvious that the differential diagnosis varies with age, e.g. osteoporosis and arthritis in the elderly, traumatic lesions in the young. In the assessment of a low back pain there are several practical tips that will be found useful: ten are listed in Box 18.1.

When it comes to severe backache in a younger person the main differential diagnosis usually lies between (1) a group of muscle and ligament 'strains', (2) disc prolapse, and (3) so-called 'apophyseal joint dysfunction'. The other conditions listed will be much further down the list. The practitioner needs a quick and useful clinical approach to the problem. Keep the 'ten practical points' as a check-list in the back of your mind in any consultation for backache. Key points in the history when considering a possible prolapsed disc will be as in Table 18.2.

You must decide whether this pain is due to an organic cause, and if so, whether it could be a disc prolapse. Remember that a mechanical pain is aggravated by movement and relieved by rest. There exists a great deal of controversy over the possible role

Table 18.1 The more common causes of a low backache

Musculoskeletal conditions	Ligamentous strain
	Muscle and other soft tissue injury
	Subluxed facet joints
	Sacroiliac strain
	Prolapsed intervertebral disc
	Fracture
	Scoliosis
Degenerative conditions	Osteoarthrosis
	Spondylosis
Rheumatic conditions	Rheumatoid arthritis
	Ankylosing spondylitis
Neoplastic conditions	Primary or secondary
Referred pain	Gynaecological
	Renal
	Other abdominal
Infection	Tuberculosis
	Osteomyelitis
	Herpes of nerve root
Psychological	Depression
	Malingering
Metabolic	Osteoporosis
	Paget's disease
	Osteomalacia

Table 18.2 History suggestive of disc prolapse

Pain: site, character, radiation	Pressure on a nerve root may give the shooting pain of sciatica. The pain may pass down the whole back of the leg or only as far as the calf
Aggravated by coughing, sneezing	Characteristic of nerve root irritation
Worse on movement, eased by rest	Mechanical back pain suggested by this
Recurrences	Common in disc prolapse
Precipitating trauma	Very often in fact no history or only of trivial trauma. Usually of sudden onset
Bowel and bladder symptoms	Any retention, recent incontinence or difficulty in micturition: This is a surgical emergency
Numbness and weakness in the legs	Corresponds to the nerve root involved
Occupation	This helps in deciding further management, e.g. time off work

Box 18.1 Ten practical tips in the assessment of a low back pain

1. Age of patient: over 50, the incidence of degenerative disease, Paget's disease and malignancy is much higher and these should be considered
2. Remember depression as a cause of low back pain
3. Is the patient generally healthy or are there signs of systemic illness, e.g. weight loss?
4. Pain at rest, morning stiffness, backache in a young person under 20, severe progressive pain, all are suspicious and merit further investigation
5. Pain that is related to posture, episodic, made worse on movement and relieved by rest is likely to be caused by a musculoskeletal condition as in Table 18.1
6. Severe limitation of straight leg raising strongly suggests lumbar disc prolapse
7. Diagnostically plain X-rays are of limited use, especially in younger patients. They may be normal in disc prolapse
8. Back pain with sciatica can occasionally be the presenting symptom of a tumour; remember the old man with carcinoma of the prostate
9. Central disc protrusion may cause bladder symptoms and this is an emergency. Ask about bladder symptoms, especially recent retention and incontinence
10. Occupation of patient. This should be asked as it helps in the management and may reveal the main reasons for consultation, i.e. compensation, certification, etc.

of apophyseal joints in the generation of back pain. It is probably impossible to diagnose the pain of apophyseal joint derangement with any degree of certainty; the history is said to be of sudden backache following a simple movement, occasionally associated with a click. Examination may reveal decreased mobility over one or more spinal segments and there is often tenderness over the spinous processes. Apophyseal joint pain does respond well to manipulation, accounting for some of the success of this technique with low backache.

How would you have examined this patient?

With experience, the way a patient comes into the room often makes the diagnosis easier. A patient who bounds into the surgery is unlikely to have a slipped disc. In this case the symptoms were typical and extensive examination was unnecessary.

Examination of the back in a patient presenting with acute back pain rarely takes more than 2–3 minutes if competently carried out (see Table 18.3).

The two roots most commonly involved are L5 and S1 (Table 18.4)

Sacroiliac strain is an occasional cause of acute low backache and these joints are worth testing (pelvic springing).

Would you have asked this patient to attend hospital for an X-ray or blood test?

Neither of these investigations is likely to be helpful in her current predicament. It would be positively unkind to ask her to attend for X-ray when in such pain, and the information yielded would be minimal. Blood tests are likely to be normal too. In the elderly, in those with suspected ankylosing spondylitis or suspected neoplasia or in those with prolonged undiagnosed back pain, an X-ray will be useful and radiographic examination is best reserved for these groups.

How would you manage this patient?

About 80% of acute backaches will resolve in 4 weeks regardless of treatment, the more minor causes disappearing sooner. The likelihood is therefore that it will resolve with conservative treatment.

The principles of treatment for such a patient will be the following.

1. Rest. A few days rest will help but the old regimen of prolonged bed rest is now out of favour—early mobilization being the aim.

2. Analgesia and relaxants. Every doctor has his own favourite analgesic for back pain and there is no shortage of choice; it must, just as in terminal care, be given *regularly* and in adequate doses. Drugs of addiction must, of course, be avoided for chronic or recurrent backache. For mild pain use simple paracetamol preparations, reserving dihydrocodeine for the more severe backache. Often diazepam in addition to paracetamol will satisfactorily control severe pain due to muscle spasm. Prescribing an anti-inflammatory is another consideration.

3. Advice. Patients must be advised on analgesia and on general back care (see later).

There is one further technique that may well have helped in the initial stage, and that is epidural injection of steroid and local anaesthetic through the sacral

Table 18.3 Examination of the back

Examination	Information obtained
Observation of the back	Acute disc prolapse: there may be a forward tilt obliterating lumbar lordosis and a lateral tilt (sciatic scoliosis)
Palpation of the back	Local tenderness common in apophyseal joint, ligamentous injury and often in acute disc prolapse. Note that acutely tender areas due to strains may be helped by local injection
Movements (flexion, extension, rotation, lateral flexion. Also test the sacroiliac joints)	In ligamentous injuries the movements are likely to be full. In apophyseal joint dysfunction there may be locally reduced mobility. In disc prolapse movements are restricted by pain but one or two movements (often flexion) restricted more than others
Straight leg raising	Reduced in prolapsed intervertebral disc with sciatic nerve irritation
Femoral stretch test (knee flexion when prone)	Positive if upper lumbar root involved
Power	In particular test movements of foot and big toe
Sensation	Especially the saddle area, as saddle area anaesthesia may be a feature of central protrusion

Table 18.4 Features of L5 and S1 root involvement

Nerve root affected	Disc involved	Straight leg raising	Ankle jerk	Weakness	Sensory loss
L5	L4/L5	↓	Present	Big toe and foot dorsiflexion	Medial side of foot (dorsum and big toe)
S1	L5/S1	↓	Absent	Plantar flexion and foot eversion	Lateral side of foot

hiatus. This requires skill in administration and will be beyond the expertise of general practitioners. If symptoms are severe and unabating and an epidural is deemed necessary the patient will invariably need to be referred to the hospital clinic.

What about manipulation and corsets?

Manipulation is a huge subject and the enthusiast can attend many courses to become proficient in the art (write to the British Association for Manipulative Medicine). If you believe apophyseal joints to be a major cause of backache then you may wish to acquire this skill; there is no doubt that manipulation can be successful in some cases. With apophyseal joint dysfunction, manipulation may involve rotation of the spine, locking the facets, and then a small jerk at the end of the manipulation. Manipulation is also useful for the minor mechanical backaches. Very important are the contraindications to manipulations, which include (1) neurological signs, e.g. major weakness, sensory loss, (2) micturition disturbances, (3) anti-coagulation, (4) radiation of pain. It thus is not appropriate in this case.

A corset helps those with mechanical back strain to stay at work and avoid recurrences.

Two days later I saw Mrs Liberty at home; the nurse had reported unsatisfactory progress. She was sitting up in bed complaining bitterly of pain. There was a nearly full bottle of tablets on her bedside table. The straight leg raising was much further reduced, the left ankle jerk absent and both legs seemed very weak. Examination showed in fact a marked deterioration. I referred her to hospital. She agreed to go, after some initial hesitation, when her husband said he would look after the home.

When would you refer a patient with backache to hospital?

1. *For diagnosis.* Unusual not to have made a diagnosis. Always remember depression and psychological causes if the diagnosis is obscure. X-rays, a few simple blood tests (including blood count and erythrocyte sedimentation rate/plasma viscosity and a sharp clinical acumen are all that is usually necessary, even in difficult cases.
2. *Suspected serious disease*, i.e. neoplasia, tuberculosis, referred pain.
3. *Treatment*, e.g. for an epidural injection.

4. *Failure of conservative therapy.*
5. *Emergency referral for surgery.* Very rarely for a cauda equina lesion as a result of massive central prolapse of an intervertebral disc. Symptoms and signs of this lesion are:
   a. saddle area anaesthesia
   b. retention of urine/urinary symptoms
   c. atonic anal sphincter
   d. severe weakness of legs peripherally.

In hospital this patient responded to rest and an epidural injection. She came home about 10 days later, still in some pain but much better than when I had last seen her. Recovery was slow, however, and she needed much reassurance and support.

Are you surprised they did not operate?

No, even with a severe prolapse the majority resolve with conservative treatment. Progression of neurological signs, cauda equina lesions and severe incapacitating pain are indications but even here the technique of chemonucleolysis—injecting the disc with chymopapain—may save the need for an operation. The technique of microdiscectomy has, however, improved prospects for patients, being a short stay procedure. Discectomy is certainly no cure for backache and is especially unwise if there is thought to be any psychological overlay to the pain.

Physiotherapy is useful after a back injury and, indeed, any patient with muscular/ligamentous backache not back to full activity within 6 weeks. Direct access to physiotherapy departments is increasingly common. Heat in its various forms, including shortwave diathermy, is soothing and physiotherapists will reinforce the back care you advise.

How would you manage this patient in the future?

Every doctor ought to have booklets on back care in the surgery which can be given to the patient. Much of this book has been devoted to the advice doctors can give patients, and backache is no exception. A few minutes of good advice can be the saving of many consultations in the future.

This lady was overweight and it was a good opportunity to encourage dieting. I also emphasized three rules:

1. Avoid lifting heavy weights, and when lifting bend at the knees, keeping the back straight.

2. Try and avoid bending the back. Sit well back in a chair rather than with your back bent. A lumbar support, e.g. a small cushion, is useful when sitting.

3. Lying rests the back. Ensure that there is a firm mattress.

There are isometric exercises the patient can be encouraged to do. In the prevention of relapses some patients are prescribed a lumbosacral belt, but judging by the ones I have seen the effect must be more psychological than physical!

A summary of acute backache management is given in Figure 18.1.

TEACHING POINTS

1. In over three-quarters of cases symptoms disappear within 4 weeks with simple analgesia alone.
2. Revise the ten practical tips in the assessment of a low back pain.
3. Learn the features of a prolapsed intervertebral disc.
4. Work out for yourself a quick efficient method for examining the back in a general practitioner's surgery.
5. Revise the reasons for referral to hospital.
6. Remember depression as a cause of backache.
7. With anyone presenting with backache, a few minutes spent in educating the patient about back care (± booklet) is good practice.

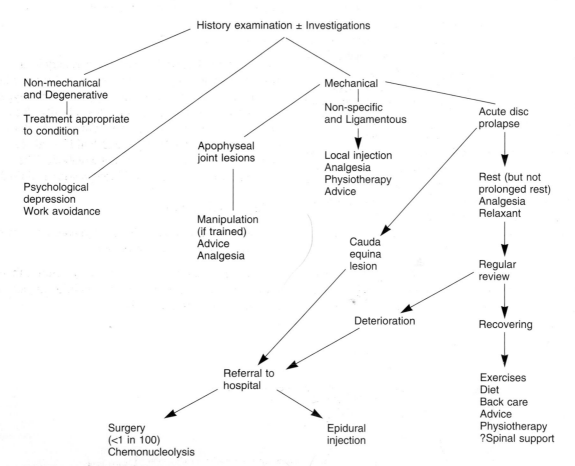

Fig. 18.1 Management of acute backache; a personal approach.

19 RISK FACTOR ASSESSMENT IN THE PREVENTION OF CORONARY ARTERY DISEASE

This chapter is concerned with the assessment of risk factors in coronary artery disease. Half the population have lipid levels above 5.8 mmol/l and one-third smoke; 6% of the population have diastolic blood pressures above 110 mmHg. There is well-documented evidence that blood pressure in the community follows a gaussian curve (Fig. 19.1). Figure 19.2 shows the increasing risk of death from hypertension. Only one person in 20 who presents with hypertension has this as the only coronary risk factor. Additional risk factors multiply the risk of coronary heart disease.

If all the present knowledge about cardiovascular disease prevention were applied, the mortality rate from this cause and the premature loss of life before the age of 65 could be reduced by a quarter.

The challenge to general practitioners is to keep abreast of developments to give optimum care to their patients. This does not necessarily mean the best that can be offered, taking into account the practical constraints of a defined population and conflicting priorities for individual patients. Hard decisions sometimes have to be made.

Mr Anstey was a 53-year-old lecturer in economics and he placed a neatly folded copy of the Guardian newspaper across his knees as he began to speak.

I'm afraid I have rather a bad family history of heart disease and I've come to ask you what the risks are for me? It was indeed a bad history: his mother died at the age of 48 from 'heart disease'; his sister died at the age of 30 from a coronary thrombosis; his brother aged 54 has angina; his father died in his 70s with some form of heart trouble.

What do you do next?

Having elicited a family history of coronary heart disease, Mr Anstey clearly needs assessing for the other major risk factors (smoking, hypertension, hypercholesterolaemia, diabetes mellitus, obesity, lack of exercise, excess alcohol intake). You find he doesn't smoke, is of average weight and build for his height and exercises regularly. He is not a diabetic. The next two steps are to measure his blood pressure and lipids.

Taking the blood pressure

Considering the diagnosis of hypertension three important points are worth noting:

1. Blood pressure has no reliable symptoms, therefore doctors should anticipate the condition in patients for whom they are responsible.

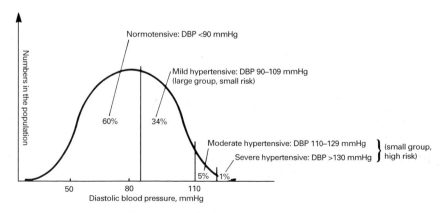

Fig. 19.1 Distribution of blood pressure levels in the community.

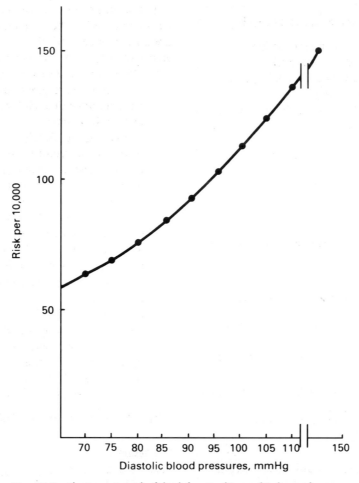

Fig. 19.2 The increasing risk of death from cardio-vascular disease for a man between the ages of 45 and 74.

2. A single reading of a patient's blood pressure, while being a fairly reliable predictor of risk, is unlikely to represent the true level of pressure—60% of patients will have a lower reading on subsequent measurement. Therefore, in order to categorize the patient satisfactorily, it is necessary to take the average of three readings on three separate occasions. This average figure is a much more reliable indicator of the value of treatment for the patient.

3. It is very important that blood pressure is recorded accurately. Box 19.1 shows sources of error in blood pressure recording.

A suggested routine is:

1. Patient in sitting position. Record with the patient sitting after a few minutes rest and the arm horizontal. Use the correct cuff size—larger cuffs for obese arms.

2. Estimate the systolic pressure first by the pressure required to stop brachial artery pulsation. Then estimate the blood pressure by placing the stethoscope over the brachial artery and inflating the cuff to 30 mmHg above the estimated systolic.

3. Record the first Korotkoff sound (the regular appearance of sounds)

4. Record the first Korotkoff sound (the disappearance of sound). If there is more than 10 mmHg between the 4th (muffling) and the 5th sound, record the 4th. A good practice is to record the 1st, 4th and 5th sounds.

1. Faulty technique, no standard routine
2. Not reading the scale at eye level
3. Terminal digit preference—rounding up to the nearest 5 or 10 mmHg
4. Inconsistent use of the 4th or 5th Korotkoff sounds
5. Variation between observers
6. Variation of the same observer at different times
7. Use of wrong size of cuff

5. Record the scale with the eyes horizontally to the nearest 2 mmHg.

Principles of managing a patient with hypertension

1. Ensure the diagnosis has been properly made on the basis of at least three readings.
2. Document other known risk factors for coronary heart disease.
3. Look for target organ damage and underlying causes by:
   a. examining the cardiovascular system
   b. examining the fundi — retinopathy
   c. testing the urine proteinuria — nephropathy
   d. measuring the urea, electrolytes and creatinine (blood glucose and lipids will also be assessed as part of 2)
   e. performing a resting ECG.

4. For all patients advise on non-pharmacological measures to reduce blood pressure (lose weight, stop smoking, reduce alcohol to <21 units (men) or <14 units (women) per week, more exercise, less salt).
5. Decide on treatment, remembering:
   a. systolic blood pressure is an independent risk and should be treated if the systolic BP is persistently >160 mmHg
   b. treating the elderly is of proven benefit; age >60 is a risk factor for hypertension
   c. a few patients give a spuriously high reading when a doctor takes their blood pressure (called 'white coat hypertension') and may benefit from ambulatory blood pressure monitoring to determine their true blood pressure.
6. The following should be treated:
   a. those with a systolic BP >160 mmHg
   b. those with a persistently elevated diastolic BP >100 mmHg
   c. for those with a diastolic BP of 90–99 mmHg, treat those over age 60, those with target organ damage (stroke, angina, cardiomegaly, retinopathy, renal failure, etc.) and those with major risk factors (diabetics, smokers, those with hyperlipidaemia or a poor family history).

The goal of treatment is <160/90 mmHg.

Drug treatment
There are a variety of antihypertensives available, each with advantages and disadvantages. Tailor treatment to the patient. The main groups are listed in Table 19.1.

Table 19.1 Main groups of antihypertensives

Group	Features	Side-effects
Thiazides	Cheap. Useful in elderly	Gout, diabetes, hyperlipidaemia, impotence, hypokalaemia
Beta-blockers	Useful for angina and postmyocardial infarction patients	Tiredness, bronchoconstriction, insomnia, lipid changes, cold peripheries, impotence, heart failure, bradycardia. Mask symptoms of hypoglycaemia
ACE inhibitors	Useful for those with heart failure, diabetes, left ventricular failure	Dry cough in about 15%. Use with caution if renal impairment. Require monitoring of renal function. Do not use with potassium-sparing diuretics. Beware using in patients with peripheral vascular disease
Angiotensin II antagonists	As effective as ACE inhibitors but without the cough	
Calcium antagonists	Useful for Afro-Caribbean patients and those with angina	Headache, flushing, ankle oedema
Alpha-blockers	Useful for those with hyperlipidaemia	Postural hypotension

Useful combinations of drugs are:

1. Diuretics + beta-blockers or ACE inhibitors.
2. Beta-blocker + diuretic or calcium antagonist or alpha-blocker. Do not use a beta-blocker with verapamil.
3. ACE inhibitor + calcium antagonist.

Monitoring
Every 3 months the blood pressure should be checked.

Referral
The following patients with hypertension merit referral to hospital: those with malignant hypertension (as an emergency); those with suspected secondary hypertension: those difficult to control: those with multiple risk factors or target organ damage; those < 35 years old.

Other risk factors

When assessing other risk factors for coronary heart disease it is useful to have a table to calculate risk and demonstrate that risk to the patient. Figure 19.3 is an example of such a risk table. Note there is a factor of 128 times the risk if a patient is a heavy smoker with a diastolic BP of 105 mmHg and a cholesterol of 7.5 mmol/l, compared with his normal counterpart.

When considering treatment of hypercholesterolaemia in particular, it is important to quantify the risk. A recent 1997 Standing Medical Advisory Committee has recommended cholesterol lowering therapy for those with a risk of a major coronary event of 3% per year (30% over 10 years).

Hyperlipidaemia

Cholesterol: who should be tested?
The ideal cholesterol is < 5.2 mmol/l. A raised cholesterol is very common. If you take a figure of 6.5 mmol/l (which doubles the risk of a myocardial infarction), a quarter of the adult UK population have cholesterol above this level. We have now major evidence of the value of treating a raised cholesterol in both secondary (patients with existing coronary heart disease, e.g. the

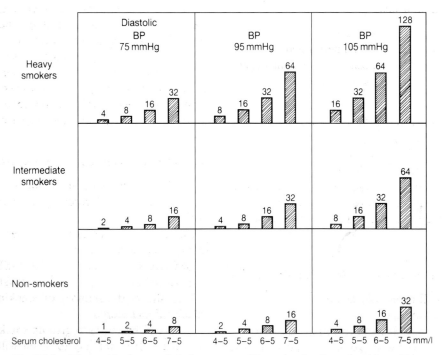

Fig. 19.3 Relative risk of myocardial infarction in middle-aged males. (Reproduced from *ACT now on cardiovascular disease. Prevention in primary care*, 1990, by permission of the Health Education Authority, London.)

> **Box 19.2** Priority target groups for lipid testing
>
> 1. All people with vascular disease under the age of 60
> 2. All patients with a family history of hyperlipidaemia
> 3. Patients with xanthoma
> 4. Patients with xanthelasma or corneal arcus under the age of 40
> 5. Patients with hypertension or diabetes mellitus
> 6. Patients undergoing coronary bypass surgery or angioplasty
> 7. Relatives (siblings or children) of patients found to have a high blood cholesterol (>7.8 mmol/l)

4S trial) and primary prevention (e.g. the WOSCOPS trial). While many patients would benefit from cholesterol lowering, it is sensible to start by screening high risk groups.

Who then should be tested?

Box 19.2 shows the primary target groups on whom a serum lipid estimation should be performed.

You need at least two readings to confirm hypercholesterolaemia. Once a raised cholesterol has been found:

1. Repeat fasting together with HDL and LDL cholesterol. Remember it is the LDL cholesterol that is the risk factor for heart disease.
2. Exclude secondary causes of hyperlipidaemia. These include obesity, alcoholism, use of certain drugs, diabetes, liver and renal failure, hypothyroidism
3. Quantify the risks to the patient by documenting other risk factors.

What should be done about a raised cholesterol?

1. Advise on all other risk factors.
2. Encourage exercise.
3. Advise on a cholesterol-lowering diet but remember that diet, even when complied with, can only reduce serum cholesterol by at most 15%. A trial of diet should be for 3–6 months.
4. Use statins (the drugs of choice for treating hypercholesterolaemia) if diet fails to lower the LDL cholesterol to < 3.2 mmol/l, if the patient has had a myocardial infarction, or < 3.4 mmol/l, if the patient has a previous history of coronary heart disease (equating to a total cholesterol of < 5.2 mmol/l). These are the main target groups for cholesterol-lowering therapy. Patients with a total cholesterol above 7.8 mmol/l will need consideration for therapy, aiming to reduce the cholesterol to ≤ 5.2 mmol/l. Patients with this high cholesterol may have familial hypercholesterolaemia and need either referral for a specialist opinion and/or screening of relatives. Patients with a cholesterol between 6.5 and 7.8 mmol/l will benefit from drug treatment if other major risk factors are present (e.g. diabetes, hypertension or a low (<0.9 mmol/l) HDL cholesterol). If a patient's cholesterol is 5.2–6.4 mmol/l, dietary advice is all that is generally required unless significant/multiple coronary heart disease risk factors are present.

Smoking

About one-quarter of all cardiovascular disease deaths are caused by smoking. On average those who die as a result of smoking lose between 10 and 15 years of life. Stopping smoking is effective. The benefits begin almost at once and those effects which are reversible will have disappeared from the statistics after 7 years.

The most cost-effective intervention is for a general practitioner to help a patient to stop smoking. Studies have shown that general practitioners advising patients to stop have success rates between 10% and 25%.

What practical steps can a doctor take?

1. Identify your smoking patients.
2. Ask about and record your patients' smoking habits.

One idea is to use an adhesive label with the following preprinted format:

SMOKER	/day	NON-SMOKER
Since 19____		Never/stopped 19____

This allows the number of smoking years to be calculated and scored.

3. Ask if they wish to give up smoking and record the answer. It is unlikely that you will be successful with someone who does not wish to stop.
4. Stress this to those who already have a smoking-related condition.

5. Offer those expressing an interest in stopping a leaflet.

6. Positively advise them to stop.

7. Offer to follow them up.

8. Write a reminder in the notes to ask next time you see them.

9. Consider a private prescription for nicotine-containing products to aid withdrawal.

How should we implement a strategy for identifying and treating risk factors for coronary artery disease?

The opportunities provided by the new contract are many:

1. new patient registrations
2. routine examination every 3 years for those not otherwise seen
3. health promotion checks
4. screening the elderly.

These are opportunities to measure the blood pressure and consider other risk factors in a large proportion of the practice population and, if combined with an opportunistic approach to those who have not had their blood pressure or other risks assessed in any other setting, make it possible to screen 95% of the practice population over a period of 5 years. Such an opportunity should not be missed and a protocol for this should be drawn up.

Taking the blood pressure is the key to targeting the high risk groups for two reasons:

1. It is the single most important and best researched risk factor.

2. It is a simple measurement and not intrusive.

A key target for screening will be those with existing coronary heart disease. Secondary prevention in this group of patients is highly cost effective and a good use of general practice resources. In particular, try to identify those with a past medical history of a myocardial infarction—are these postinfarction patients:

- still smoking?
- on aspirin?
- on a beta-blocker?
- on an ACE inhibitor?
- assessed for hypercholesterolaemia and, if required (see chest pain chapter), treated with a statin?
- controlled in respect of hypertension?

An audit of patients post myocardial infarction is a valuable exercise and can be practice nurse led.

TEACHING POINTS

1. The assessment of cardiovascular risk factors is a logical way of identifying those who are at greatest risk of developing coronary thrombosis.
2. There are simple steps that a general practitioner, can take to identify and reduce the most important risk factors for an individual patient.
3. A practice population can be monitored and the benefits can be demonstrated although individual patients may choose not to co-operate.
4. It is important to fully understand and implement the evidence-based management of patients with hypertension and hyperlipidaemia.

20 VAGINAL DISCHARGE

Vaginal discharge is a common symptom during a woman's fertile years. The majority of women will experience vaginitis at some time in their lives. It can occur at any age and such discharges occurring outside the reproductive years should be viewed with special care. Discharge can be affected by menstruation, oral contraceptives, age, pregnancy and sexual activity. Accurate diagnosis and effective treatments are important to a woman's sexual health.

Chlamydia is the most prevalent sexually transmitted disease in the western world. In 50% of cases women are asymptomatic. Boxes 20.1 and 20.2 list the causes of vaginal discharge and acute pruritus vulvae.

Box 20.1 Causes of vaginal discharge in descending order of frequency

- Excessive normal secretions
- Infection: candidiasis, bacterial vaginosis, trichomoniasis
- Cervicitis (gonococcal, chlamydial, herpetic)
- Cervical ectropion (erosion)
- Cervical polyp
- Foreign body (e.g. lost tampon, ring pessary, or other items)
- Intrauterine contraceptive device
- Bartholinitis
- Neoplasia: (1) vulvo vaginal; (2) cervical or uterine
- Sloughing intrauterine fibroid
- Pyometria
- Pelvic fistula

Box 20.2 Causes of acute pruritis vulvae

- Vaginal candidiasis
- Herpes simplex
- Contact dermatitis or allergies

The cornerstones of accurate diagnosis are:

1. a good history
2. the appropriate examination
3. microbiological tests.

Treatment can usually be supervised by the general practitioner but if the discharge is stubbornly recurrent or related to risk factors for sexually transmitted diseases then referral to a genitourinary medical (GUM) clinic is advisable.

Vivienne Cato is a 21-year-old student, recently married, who came to my surgery requesting pessaries to clear up a discharge she had had for the last week. She had had two visits in the last 8 months for the same symptom and on each occasion had been given Canesten pessaries. On the first occasion one of the partners had sent off a high vaginal swab which had grown Candida albicans. She also complained of severe itching 'in the front passage'. Pessaries had helped last time but she further volunteered that she had never really been clear of the discharge for the last 2 months, since the last course of pessaries.

What questions would you would ask her?

The first question I asked in fact was, what she thought the cause might be and whether she thought it was similar in nature to the discharge she had had when we had isolated *Candida*. She replied, she thought she had 'thrush' and the discharge was similar to that experienced before.

There are many questions you could ask in elucidating the cause of a vaginal discharge and a summary appears in Box 20.3. Of particular importance is the nature of the discharge, relation to periods, the use of drugs, including contraceptives, and a history of sexual contacts where appropriate.

The general practitioner should try to discover the

patient's idea of causation: it may well reveal a fear
of disease that is the real reason for the consultation.
A doctor's knowledge of the patient will help when
considering psychological causes, but a careful examination at least once must be considered. In at least
half of all the cases of vaginal discharge which you
will see in practice, no cause will be found, and in
some of these it will be the patient who perceives a
normal secretion as an 'abnormal vaginal discharge'.

The date of the last menstrual period may seem an
odd question to the patient, but occasionally an un-
suspected pregnancy will be detected. It is to be hoped
that all doctors will know whether their patients are
taking antibiotics, contraceptives, etc., but this should
be checked. Questioning about sexual contacts is not
as difficult as it sounds and will obviously be important; a gentle and tactful approach is needed. Although
the possibility of serious sexually transmitted disease,
i.e. gonorrhoea or syphilis, must be considered, it is
comparatively rare in an average practice. If strongly
suspected, the patient is best referred to a genitourinary department for full investigation, treatment,
follow-up and contact tracing. A past history will
obviously increase suspicion on this score. It may
of course be neither easy nor tactful to suggest that
you wish to exclude venereal disease. A helpful
approach is to explain that the discharge may not be
easy to investigate in the context of the surgery and
that hospitals are better able to help in this situation.
If this suggestion is unacceptable the appropriate
swabs should be taken in your surgery.

Candidiasis normally presents as a creamy white,
cheesy, itchy discharge.

Bacterial vaginosis (BV) presents with a grey non-
purulent discharge characterized by an offensive fishy
smell. Risk factors for BV include vaginal douching,
use of the intrauterine contraceptive device and many
sexual partners.

Trichomonas vaginalis produces an offensive
yellowish/greenish/purulent discharge, possibly itchy,
with a vulval soreness and painful vaginitis.

*She had in fact been married for 9 months, to her
first and only boy-friend. Since the age of 18 she
had been using oral contraception.*

*What examination or investigations would you have
carried out?*

It is important in treating vaginal discharge to make
as accurate a diagnosis as possible and this means
a careful examination. This principle is even more
important with a recurrent discharge. The prescription
of drugs and pessaries without examination may well
lead to disappointment by both patient and doctor.
Just as important is a negative finding, i.e. no cause
found, and this may mean that psychological factors
have been missed.

The patient's response to the suggestion that an
examination may be necessary is often an important
clue to the problem. If she appears distressed or
reluctant, this is the opportunity to say 'You seem to
be unhappy about an examination …'; an open-ended
statement often allows the patient to express some
of her misgivings, which can be an important clue
to her thoughts about the problem. The sight of a
speculum is frequently alarming to the patient and
it is often wiser to perform a bimanual examination
first, followed by the gentle insertion of a speculum.
A gentle and sympathetic approach is particularly
necessary when the patient has never been examined
before.

In this case I examined the vulva before the insertion of a sterile Cusco's speculum. Erythema and
fissuring are the most common findings in candidiasis.
A speculum examination is valuable for a variety of
reasons; it often establishes the cause of a discharge—
the discharge can be seen and swabs taken, foreign
bodies, erosions and polyps can be identified. During
vaginal examination look for the thick white adherent

plaques classic of candidiasis. Look also at the cervix. A mucopurulent discharge from the os indicates cervicitis. Bimanual examination (useful where pregnancy or pelvic inflammation is suspected) completes the examination.

I noticed that Mrs Cato had thick white patches of discharge on the vaginal walls and I took a high vaginal swab; the appearances were typical of Candida infection. The cervix showed a mild erosion.

Investigations

Table 20.1 shows the investigations possible in a case of a vaginal discharge.

Candidiasis can be detected with a high vaginal swab, and infection with *Trichomonas vaginalis* by means of a wet smear or by culture; most laboratories have their own trichomonal transport medium and practitioners may request a supply.

It is easy to forget gonorrhoea. For the precise diagnosis, swabs from the cervix, urethra and rectum are required. The most likely site to yield a positive result is the endocervix. First visualize the cervix with a sterile speculum and wash the mucus plug off with a swab dipped in sterile water. Using a charcoal swab a specimen can then be taken from just within the cervical canal. The swab should be put straight into Stuart's transport medium and sent to the laboratory. Stuart's transport medium may in fact only preserve enough gonococci for diagnosis for 24 hours so that

speed in transport is essential. At the same time a urethral swab may be sent. If facilities are available an immediate smear and Gram stain will give results, but this is not always easy and is beyond the experience of the average practitioner. If you are taking swabs for suspected gonorrhoea the patient ought to be referred to a genitourinary department, as contact tracing, follow-up, etc. will be required. Remember, gonorrhoea and trichomoniasis often coexist, so that often the trichomonal discharge is treated, missing the gonorrhoea. With a suspicious history or the sight of pus issuing from the cervix, refer.

In this case the history and physical signs suggested *Candida*. I took a high vaginal swab to confirm my clinical impression in view of the persistence of the discharge. She had had a smear recently as part of her contraception follow-up. Since this was becoming a recurrent problem I tested the urine and it was negative. With no history of more than one contact and with typical symptoms and signs of candidiasis I did not take swabs for gonorrhoea or refer.

What is the probable cause of this patient's discharge?

Candidiasis is, of course, the most likely cause of this patient's discharge. Fry has estimated that in about one-third of cases *Candida* is the cause of a vaginal discharge (7% being due to *Trichomonas vaginalis*, and in over half no cause being found). It is commonly associated with pruritus vulvae and often recurrent. *Candida* may flourish due to some underlying reason, notably diabetes, pregnancy, steroids, candidiasis in the sexual partner, and the use of antibiotics.

When might you consider referring a patient with a vaginal discharge?

Referral for the symptom of vaginal discharge is usually confined to four areas:

1. suspected venereal disease
2. repeated recurrence of unknown cause
3. abnormal cytology or suspected malignancy
4. cervical erosions or polyps—but beware attributing the cause to them.

The role of chlamydia infection (causing a cervicitis with a secondary discharge) has been highlighted and if this is suspected (i.e. the patient has a cervicitis

Table 20.1 Investigation of a vaginal discharge

Investigation	Organism isolated
1. High vaginal swab	BV, candida, trichomonas
2. Vaginal pH (measured with standard pH paper)	< or = 4.5: normal, candida >4.5: BV, trichomonas
3. Microscopic examination of wet smear	'Clue cells' shown in BV; motile trichomonads seen in trichomonas infection
4. Endocervical swab	Chlamydia, gonococcus
5. Whiff test (drop of potassium hydroxide added to vaginal secretion)	Produces a fishy smell with BV

DNA amplification testing of first catch urine specimen most acceptable diagnosis for chlamydia. Candida and trichomonas may be detected on a cervical smear.

or the male partner has a urethritis), the patient may be best referred. Gonorrhoea has also been mentioned; remember that it is asymptomatic in over half of the women infected and salpingitis is a serious sequel; it should be considered in sexually active women with persistent or recurrent symptoms.

Always be aware of the possibility of a malignancy. In general, a blood-stained discharge tends to be associated with malignancy or pregnancy (threatened abortion, retained products, etc.), but it may just indicate a severe infection. A malignancy may, however, present merely as a foul discharge. In the postmenopausal patient any bleeding must be assumed to be due to malignancy until proved otherwise: it is a case for referral.

Finally a word about cervical erosions. These are extremely common, especially in those on the contraceptive pill, and are to a large extent asymptomatic. A vaginal discharge should not be assumed to be due to the erosion when an erosion is present, and although one large study (Goldacre et al *BMJ* March 1978) did demonstrate some association between the presence of vaginal discharge and cervical erosions, albeit a modest one, they themselves recommended that 'even when an erosion is found in a woman with abnormal discharge it should not necessarily be regarded as the cause of the discharge'. Hence, you must exclude all other causes before attributing a discharge to an erosion; take a cervical smear before referring for cryocautery. Erosions by themselves usually need no treatment.

In this case the diagnosis of candidiasis was confirmed by a high vaginal swab.

This patient has come for some pessaries to cure her 'thrush'. What preparations are available to treat candidiasis?

There are both local and oral treatments available. As with any illness advice is valuable (see below). There are several alternative local preparations; all are effective. Two of use are:

1. *Clotrimazole (Canesten) vaginal tablets and cream.* Dose: 100 mg tablet inserted nightly for 6 nights or a single 500 mg (Canesten 1) pessary inserted at night. The single pessary is particularly appreciated by patients.

2. *Miconazole (Gyno-Daktarin) pessaries, cream and tampons.* Dose: two pessaries inserted high in the vagina for 7 consecutive nights or one tampon inserted high in the vagina night and morning for 5 consecutive days or, as with Canesten, a single Gyno-Daktarin 1 pessary inserted vaginally at night.

Pessaries and creams have, until recently, been the mainstay of treatment but now a single fluconazole (Diflucan) tablet taken orally is used increasingly—it can be highly effective! Itraconazole (Sporanox) is an alternative.

What would be your strategy in a case similar to this where recurrent candidiasis is not responding to courses of pessaries?

Recurrent candidiasis due to *Candida albicans* can be difficult to treat but attention should be paid to the following.

1. *Exclude other yeasts* such as *Candida glabrata* and *Saccharomyces cerevisiae*, which can be less sensitive to antifungals.

2. *Are there any predisposing causes?* We have mentioned these. She was not on antibiotics or steroids but was using the contraceptive pill. Evidence does not support the contraceptive pill as being a precipitating factor. She had no glycosuria and the erosion is probably non-contributory. Iron deficiency is a predisposing factor and this may be worth considering.

3. *Hygiene, clothing, etc.* There is certain advice that should be given to patients with recurrent candidiasis.
a. Avoid nylon tights and pants (because of the humidity they cause).
b. Keep the vulva as cool, dry and clean as possible.
c. After defecation wipe from front to back, not vice versa.
d. Keep nails well cut and clean.

4. *Initiate prophylactic therapy.* Intermittent oral or topical treatment can be given monthly for 6 months pre- or postmenstrually, according to the patient's symptoms. Alternatively, use single-dose pessary treatment weekly for 4 weeks.

Additional notes on the management of vaginal discharge

• Vaginal candidiasis is one of the most common infections seen in general practice.
• Vaginal candidiasis affects 75% of women; 40–50% have recurrent episodes.

- *Candida albicans* accounts for 90% of episodes, *C. glabrata* for 5%.
- Vaginal candidiasis is much more common in pregnant women. A large proportion of patients with chronic recurrent candidiasis first present with the infection in pregnancy.
- Trichomoniasis can be treated by metronidazole (Flagyl) 400 mg b.d. for 7 days. Treat the partner. Warn about the effects of alcohol. Remember gonorrhoea is associated.
- The treatment of BV is metronidazole 400 mg b.d. for 7 days. Topical metronidazole gel and clindamycin cream are alternatives.

TEACHING POINTS

1. Some patients presenting with vaginal discharge will have complex fears and psychosexual or psychological difficulties.
2. Remember gonorrhoea—if suspected the patient is best referred.
3. The most common identifiable cause in general practice is candidiasis.
4. A good history and examination plus vaginal pH enables a provisional diagnosis to be made in most cases.
5. A genital tract infection can be caused by more than one pathogen.

21 FEBRILE CONVULSIONS

Febrile convulsions are 'Seizures that are provoked by fever of extracranial origin.' Three per cent of all children can expect to have a febrile convulsion between the ages of 6 months and 5 years. Only one-third can expect to have a recurrence. The average general practitioner has 10–15 patients of all ages with convulsions consulting in a year. Prophylactic treatment is controversial.

The prevalence of epilepsy up to the age of 23 is 8.4 per 1000 and in adults 5–10 per 1000; this translates into 145 000 children and 420 000 adults in the UK. One-third have generalized siezures; in one-quarter of these the onset is related to specific conditions. One in eight are prescribed a drug for 6 or more years after the last siezure (Kurtz et al 1998). Of 124 young persons in this study, six died after the age of 16 and 46 had neurological impairment or other serious health problems.

Mrs Elizabeth Newland is 6 months pregnant and sees you regularly in the antenatal clinic. She sends for you one evening because her daughter Caroline, aged 4, has had a 'funny turn'.

What questions would you ask?

A careful history is important at this stage to get a clear picture of what is being described.

Mrs Newland tells you that Caroline, while watching television, seemed to lose interest in the programme and then began to shake. She stopped and continued to watch the programme with a leaden look in her eye. 'She seems all right now', her mother adds.

Your questions should now be directed to obtaining as much information as possible about the occurrence.

- Did the mother witness the attack?
- Was there any warning that it was coming?
- Did the girl make any unusual noises?

- When she twitched, was it the whole of her body, or only part of her body?
- How long did it last?
- Did she go blue?
- Has she been incontinent?
- Did she bite her tongue?
- Has she ever had anything like this before?
- Is there any family history of blackouts?
- Has she had any previous illness, or been in contact with any infectious disease?

In answer to these questions, Mrs Newland describes the attack exactly as before. 'It lasted quite a long time.' There is no other additional information. The mother was watching her at the time and she remembered that she had a similar attack 2 years ago with a viral illness.

What problems does this pose?

From the history it is fairly clear that the girl has had a convulsion. You are not at present able to determine whether or not it is associated with a febrile illness.

What examination will you make?

A general examination reveals that Caroline is still rather sleepy and not really interested in television programmes, or in your arrival. She is conscious and cooperates but does not talk to you spontaneously. She is a normally developed, healthy-looking 4-year-old. She is about to go to nursery school and appears to be an intelligent little girl.

Examination will be directed to discovering whether there are signs of intercurrent infection, the presence of which would be a reasonable explanation for the present episode. Specifically, meningitis should be positively excluded. Look for evidence of tonsillitis and otitis media, for chest infection and to see whether she is pyrexial. Unless there has been prolonged convulsion, it is unlikely that a high temperature will be the result of muscular activity. However, in many febrile conditions, the febrile convulsions precede the pyrexia by a few hours, and the absence of a temperature does not exclude an infective cause.

How do you manage a febrile convulsion in the home?

Education and support for the parents is necessary because most parents witnessing a first convulsion think their child is dying. Management is summarized in Box 21.1. Half of all the cases of status epilepticus take place with the first fit, and phenobarbitone has little part to play in its management. Diazepam is clearly now the drug of choice for managing a convulsion and its administration has been simplified by the availability of Stesolid rectal tubes (diazepam 2 mg/ml, rectal tubes of 2.5 ml contain 5 mg diazepam)—which should be part of every general practitioner's emergency bag! In an emergency, if a rectal tube is not available the contents of an ampoule of diazepam for injection can be administered rectally.

The current view is that, in a perfect world, everyone who has a fit should be seen by a neurologist but there are not sufficient neurologists to make this

---

Box 21.1   The management of a febrile fit

1. Ensure that the airway is clear and that the child is in the left lateral position with head down (the recovery position)
2. Is the child still fitting? If so, rectal diazepam (Stesolid) is the drug of choice, and this will be given in the following dose: The dose for a child aged 1–3 is 5 mg; for those over 3 years the dose is 10 mg. This can be repeated if necessary in five minutes.
3. Reduce the fever by taking off extra clothes and blankets, giving plenty of fluids and tepid sponging. An electric fan is also helpful. Paracetamol suspension (Calpol) is the drug of choice as an antipyretic. The dose for those aged 1–5 years is 10 ml (240 mg paracetamol) 4 times daily.
4. Look for causes of the fit
5. Advise parents what to do next
6. Sodium valproate can reduce the recurrence rate but is not often used

---

possible. However, first seizures should be referred for full evaluation and management.

In this case you discover that Caroline has a slightly red throat, with no other abnormal physical signs.

What now is your plan of management?

Classification of fits and the role of prophylactic treatment

Febrile convulsions are divided into two groups, simple and complex. A simple febrile convulsion has these features:

1. It occurs in an infant developing normally aged between 1 and 5.
2. It has no focal features.
3. The fit lasts for less than 15 minutes and is generalized tonic or clonic. Family history is positive in 30–50% of cases.

In a collaborative study, no patient with a simple febrile convulsion was found to have serious subsequent neurological disorder or intellectual impairment. Only 2.2% of children with simple febrile convulsions will eventually develop convulsions without fever, and adequate prophylaxis in this group will not decrease the risk. Children with simple convulsions comprise two-thirds of all children with convulsions. Only one-third of children who have had a simple febrile convulsion will have another attack, but 10% will have multiple episodes. Figure 21.1 summarizes the statistics of febrile convulsions.

At this stage it would be wise to enquire about Caroline's birth and whether it involved a forceps delivery, and whether the perinatal period was normal. In the absence of any stronger evidence, it is reasonable to assume that this is a recurrent simple convulsion.

A complex convulsion has the following features:

1. focal signs
2. duration over 15 minutes
3. onset before the age of one
4. a family history of febrile seizures.

These children have a 10% chance of developing convulsions without fever, including temporal lobe epilepsy.

Definitions of types of epilepsy

Generalized seizures

- An absence: the person looks blank, is oblivious

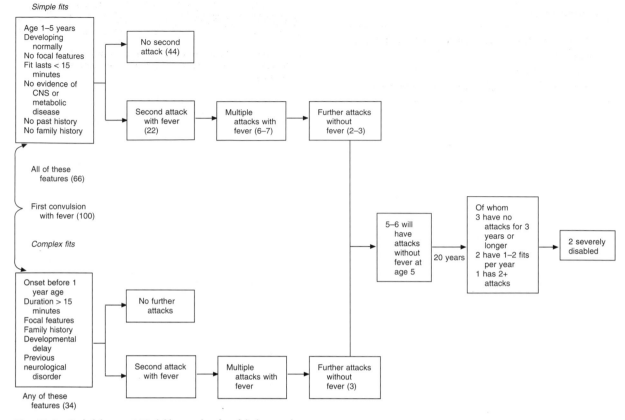

Fig. 21.1 Probabilities in 100 children with a first febrile convulsion

to external stimuli and carries on normally afterwards, often unaware that anything is amiss.
- Atonic seizures: the body loses all muscle tone and goes floppy.
- Tonic seizures: the whole body stiffens as muscles tighten.
- Tonic/clonic seizures: the body stiffens then muscles convulse.

Partial seizures
- Simple partial: slight tingling or twitching in an isolated part of the body; experience of strange tastes or smells; no loss of consciousness. These may be the precursor of other types of seizures.
- Complex partial: may include impaired consciousness, disorientation, confusion, strange behaviour, strong emotional states, confused meaningless speech.
- Secondary generalization: brain activity is partial initially but then becomes generalized.

How would you talk to Mrs Newland?

You have the advantage of an established relationship as she is seeing you in your antenatal clinic. At this stage you can say that Caroline appears to have had another febrile convulsion, this time associated with a sore throat. Because it is the second time she has had one you think that it would be wise to give her some treatment for her infection (syr. penicillin V 125 mg q.d.s. for 1 week).

There is a slight possibility that a third attack may occur. If this is the case, treatment is available to suppress further episodes. Under these circumstances you would recommend seeking a consultant opinion.

If the mother raises the question of epilepsy it is reasonable to say that there is no strong evidence which points in that direction but the possibility exists.

Your aim should be to keep this explanation at as simple a level as the circumstances and your relationship with Mrs Newland will permit. Further explanations, support and encouragement may be needed but should be deferred unless you are specifically questioned.

TEACHING POINTS

1. The history is the most important guide to the nature of a convulsion.
2. Distinguish between simple and complex fits.
3. Refer first seizures for full evaluation and management.

FURTHER READING

Kurtz Z, Tookey P, Ross E 1988 Epilepsy in young people: 23 year followup of the British national child development study. *BMJ* 316:339–342

22 CHILD ABUSE

The abuse of children, also known as 'non-accidental injury', is an increasingly recognized problem. The really severe cases make both local and national news headlines and it has been estimated that about 100 children die each year as a result. This, however, is only the tip of an iceberg; many more will suffer neurological and mental handicap and many thousands suffer minor injuries. The injury to the child's emotional development is impossible to quantify, and if one includes neglect as well as physical injury the problem becomes a very sizeable one.

There is a great problem of definition. Children are naturally apt to be 'naughty' and are also very accident prone. The family practitioner must be aware of the implications of labelling parents as 'child abusers', with the attendant stigma this will put on the parents, and it will severely jeopardize the doctor–patient relationship. The problem is in reality not as dramatic as it sounds, as by the time a diagnosis of child abuse has been made, social workers, health visitors and the doctor are all usually already involved in helping these families; it must, however, be remembered that child abuse can occur in all sorts of families with parents from all walks of life.

In this chapter we hope to familiarize readers with all aspects of child abuse, as the family practitioner is a key person in its detection and management. At all times we must remember that the child is also our patient and it is our duty to protect his or her physical and emotional development if these are severely at risk. It is only too poignantly obvious that a missed case of child abuse may be just as serious as a missed case of meningitis.

Here is a typical but fictitious case.

It concerns Gary, the 19-month-old son of a 20-year-old unemployed labourer who had been married a year. His mother, Vera, had just given birth to another son at the age of 17. John, the father, has had a turbulent childhood and had himself been subject to a Care Order and had a police record of two criminal offences. The family has a regular social worker and health visitor and is deeply in debt. The father has had alcohol problems in the past and is prone to outbursts of violence. Vera also had an unsettled childhood and had given the health visitor some concern in her casual attitude to the birth of her new son.

The family is therefore already well known to the practice. The first sign of suspected child abuse came when the midwife on a routine visit had noticed severe bruising on the older boy's cheek; the parents explained that he had fallen on to a chair. A month later he was brought twice to the surgery for treatment of a cough and I noted fresh bruises to the face. While I was undressing him, ostensibly to find the cause of the cough, the mother was reluctant for too much exposure of the boy's body. I noted, however, two unusual marks on his back and what could well have been a human bite mark on his arm.

Before continuing the story it is worth testing your current knowledge about child abuse.

Are there any indications in the parental history to predict a higher child abuse rate in these families?

Yes, there are and they are listed in Box 22.1. The case has several of the features and is therefore a 'high risk' family.

This list will thus help in defining those parents and children particularly at risk of abusing or being abused, although it must be remembered that this can occur in all families.

What different sorts of child abuse are there?

It is relatively common to think of child abuse in terms of unexplained bruises and fractures on a child, but doctors should also be aware of other forms of abuse, such as sexual abuse and failure to thrive due to

Box 22.1   Which parents? Which children?

There are many factors correlating with subsequent child abuse. The tendency for one set of parents to ill-treat their children and these children in turn to ill-treat theirs is part of the so-called 'cycle of deprivation'

Parents
Factors correlating with later child abuse include:

1. Parents are often young with little experience of child-rearing
2. The mother's pregnancy is often unwanted and there may have been a request for termination earlier in the pregnancy
3. The parents themselves may have been ill-treated as children
4. They often lack family support
5. There may be additional stress with unemployment, poor housing, poverty, alcoholism
6. Most evidence suggests higher prevalence in lower social class
7. Often frequent surgery attenders ('a cry for help')
8. Father away from home; mother not living with natural father
9. Personality; a few are aggressive and/or seriously psychiatrically ill
10. A severe puerperal depression may be present

Child
1. Most common before the child is walking and talking
2. Premature birth associated with twice the risk of abuse
3. Early separation from mother predisposes to later abuse
4. Any physical and mental defects in the child

Box 22.2   Identifying child abuse

- Always listen to the child—especially what is said spontaneously
- Be wary of delay in seeking help by the carers
- Be wary of vague explanations lacking detail
- Make notes of inappropriate responses from carers
- Is there any history of unexplained injury or illness

Indicators of physical abuse
- Bruises
    to eyes/mouth/ears
    fingertip bruises (grasp marks)
    bruises of different ages in same place
    bruises without obvious verifiable explanations
    bruises to non-mobile babies
- Burns, bites, scars
    clear impressions of teeth (more than 3 cm across likely to be adult)
    burns or scalds with clear outlines
    small round burns (cigarettes?)
    large numbers of different aged scars
    unusual shaped scars
    scars that suggest medical treatment was not received
- Fractures
    in children under 1 year
    alleged unnoticed fractures (difficult area)
- Other injuries
    poisoning, injections or application of other damaging substances
    female genital mutilation including female circumcision

Indicators of neglect
- Not receiving adequate food consistent with their potential growth
- Exposed through lack of supervision to injury or toxic dangers
- Left in circumstances likely to endanger without adult supervision
- Prevention by carer from receiving appropriate medical advice or treatment

Indicators of sexual abuse
- Sexually transmitted disease

persistent neglect; both are more common than often realized. Poisoning is more difficult to prove, as children are prone to ingest tablets anyway. The types of child abuse are shown in Box 22.2.

Looking at Box 22.2 it is obvious that the key to detection of child abuse lies in an index of suspicion over a wide spectrum of presentations of childhood

Box 22.2 (*contd*)

- Recurring urinary infection
- Genital and rectal itching and soreness
- Unexplained bleeding and discharge
- Bruising in the genital region
- Sexual play judged inappropriate to child's age, development, circumstance
- Sexually explicit behaviour
- Young children with a lot of sexual knowledge
- Sexually abusive behaviour towards other children, particularly those younger or more vulnerable
- Unexplained pregnancy

Indicators of emotional abuse
- Abnormal passive, lethargic or attention-seeking behaviour
- Specific habit disorders, e.g. faecal smearing, etc.
- Excessive nervous behaviour such as rocking or hair twisting

Box 22.3 Points to look for in the history

1. Explanation inconsistent with the injuries evident on the child
2. Discrepancies in the history; either discrepancies between parents or discrepancies between the initial and later story by the same parent
3. Previous history of child abuse or unexplained injury
4. Delayed presentation—late in seeking medical help
5. Parent may actually volunteer a fear of hitting the child
6. Inappropriate reaction to the child's injury; abnormal concern or an abnormally unconcerned attitude
7. History of repeated consultations for minor problems
8. Child brought to the surgery for another reason and injury noted
9. A reluctance to allow a full examination of the child

accidents and illness. It will be noticed that at the end of the list is the term 'emotional abuse'; repeated verbal abuse can be extremely detrimental to a child's development.

What points are there to be sought in the history when considering possible child abuse?

Always faithfully record the parents' explanation of the injuries and their reaction to them; as in all medical practice the keeping of precise written records is essential. With tact a history can usually be obtained and a direct challenge is not helpful; if the injuries are at all serious the police will also be questioning the parents on intent. Box 22.3 lists the main points in the history.

The explanation of the injury is obviously of importance and it should be possible to look for three sorts of inadequate explanation: (1) the child may not be developmentally capable of what he was supposed to have been doing, e.g. a history of climbing on to a high sideboard at 12 months; (2) the explanation may be inconsistent with respect to time, i.e. the presence of old bruises explained by a fall that morning; (3) the

explanation may be inconsistent in respect of the degree of trauma produced, e.g. massive bruising of the face explained by a fall on the living room floor.

What are the key features to be found on examination?

These are shown in Figure 22.1. The reader must be familiar in particular with some of the following characteristics:

1. *Bruising.* Finger-tip bruises are small and round, occurring together. They are often around the mouth where the parent had tried to close the child's mouth. Always note bruising of varying ages. Facial bruising is not too common accidentally, especially when it is large and on both sides of the face; this also applies to two 'black eyes'. Note bruising around the ears.

2. *Subdural haematoma.* Remember subdural haematoma—it may be very serious and is often missed.

3. *Fractures.* Normal children do sustain fractures. X-ray appearances may be highly suggestive of abuse, e.g. multiple injuries, old as well as new fractures.

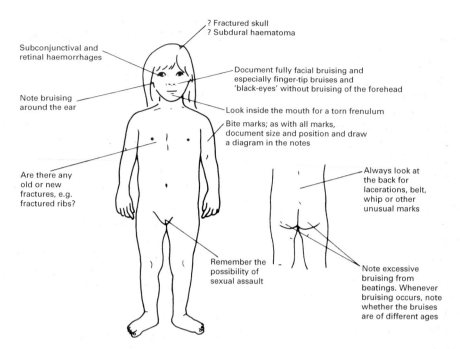

Fig. 22.1 Key features on examining a child suspected of having been abused. Look also for obvious signs of neglect, failure to thrive and retardation, particularly in the fields of communication and social interaction.

4. *Retinal haemorrhage*. This can occur due to excessive shaking of the child.

5. *Torn lip and torn frenulum*. Open the mouth to look for a torn frenulum.

6. *Burns and scalds*. Especially recognize cigarette burns.

7. *Other marks, including bites*. Be able to recognize human bite marks—semicircular bruises with imprints of teeth marks. Occasionally they will be caused by the dog, as often claimed, but they are then readily distinguished. Beware of any unusual marks—they may be of instruments used to beat a child. I recall one case with a burn neatly outlining the pointed end of an iron.

All injuries should be documented with size and position noted; this usually occurs in hospital but it is essential for all doctors to recognize the above signs of injury. A brief development assessment and a plotting of the child's height and weight are useful. It may be necessary to examine the genitals fully at some stage.

A word on investigation. A skeletal survey for old fractures is usually performed in hospital. Every case

of extensive bruising should have a full clotting screen.

Gary is in your surgery. What would be your course of action?

We have good clinical grounds for suspecting child abuse in his case (previous severe bruising, current bruising with inadequate explanation, unusual marks to the back and a bite mark). Every doctor has his own approach to child abuse, evaluating the risk of this child with these parents. In mild cases with the initial presentation of minor injury all that may be needed is the mobilization of support for the family, with monitoring of that family by health visitor and social worker. There can be few families, particularly those with the addition of other stresses such as poor housing, unemployment and poverty, who have not at any time hit their children. The challenge is really in the monitoring of these families to detect persistent abuse. All that may be needed to help some families is the continued availability and guidance of one of the members of the practice team. Occasionally an

NSPCC worker will help. Team-work and good communications are the basis of good management. There is now an on call team which can be contacted via the local hospital.

Referral to hospital is indicated for children who have received moderate or severe abuse, a sexual assault, persistent abuse, or where you are unhappy that you may not prevent further serious abuse by monitoring the situation. A further area of referral is those children with signs of serious neglect and failure to thrive.

Referral to hospital is not too difficult as a parent will usually agree to having the child 'investigated' for bruising. The advantages of hospital referral are many:

1. They will be able to carry out easily the necessary clotting screen and skeletal survey.

2. Documentation of the injuries is easier, perhaps including photographs.

3. Skilled assessment may be needed in some cases, e.g. sexual assault.

4. The injury itself may need special treatment.

5. Hospital may sometimes be a place of safety for the child.

In this case I did refer Gary to hospital with a covering letter for the paediatrician, lodged with the social worker who accompanied the boy and his mother. Note that a good covering letter or, if not practical telephone conversation is essential.

When he was admitted to the hospital ward considerable evidence of severe abuse was noted; much more than I had realized. The local Community Medical Officer was contacted and the child's injuries were documented thoroughly. They feared he would be removed from hospital, and an 'Emergency Protection Order' was obtained to prevent this while investigations were proceeding. A case conference was called.

What is a case conference, who is present and what decisions are likely?

A case conference is usually called on behalf of the appropriate Director of Social Services. Its aim is to inform all workers involved with the case and to establish cooperation between them all in further management decisions about the child's and family's future. It is thus held in only the more severe cases

> **Box 22.4** Categories of abuse for registration
>
> - Physical injury—actual or likely injury to a child
> - Neglect—persistent or severe neglect or failure to protect a child from any kind of danger
> - Sexual abuse—actual or likely sexual exploitation of a child or adolescent abuse

of child abuse. The family practitioner, as a key professional, will be invited to attend (Box 22.4).

At a typical case conference there will be:

- a hospital paediatrician dealing with the case
- the family practitioner
- the community medical officer dealing with the case
- the social worker
- the health visitor
- a police officer
- a more senior social worker
- the local authority's solicitor (for legal advice)
- a secretary (to document the discussion).

There are various decisions to be taken following a full discussion between the interested parties of the home background, the history, the clinical findings, relevant past history, etc., each individual adding a particular part to the whole. There are two basic processes:

1. The child is placed on the local Child Protection Register (Box 22.5). Since if one child in a family has been abused the other is clearly at risk, both this child's name and that of his baby brother will have been put on the Register. The Register has several uses, in that, when dealing with a child suspected of having been subject to abuse, suspicions may be heightened if the child is on the Register. In our area the local Casualty Department has a copy of the Register. The Register provides statistics useful in monitoring care and helps to ensure follow-up on certain families. The Register is reviewed regularly, with people being added to and removed from it. The problem of confidentiality is a thorny one.

2. The decision to be made is whether proceedings should be taken to the juvenile court and if so (i.e. if

Box 22.5 The Child Protection Register

- *The register maintains*:
  A record of all children who are subject to an interagency protection plan
  A record of enquiries made about children in the last 3 years
- *Criteria for placing a child's name on the register*:
  That, following a child protection conference, there must have been identified reasons or incidents having adversely affected the child. It is important to identify a specific occasion when harm has occurred or professional judgement that harm is likely. An interagency plan is necessary

These guidelines are produced by the Leicestershire and Rutland Area Child Protection Committee

8 days, with a possible extension of 7 days) have replaced 'Place of Safety Orders' and parents have the right to challenge this order only 72 hours after it has been instituted. A court can still make a Care Order (the child being placed in the care of the local authority) or a Supervision Order (whereby the child is allowed home under the supervision of an officer—usually a social worker). These orders can only be made if the court is satisfied that a child has suffered, or is likely to suffer, significant abuse and this suffering is a result of a neglect of the standard of care one would expect from a parent of a similar child (or as a result of the child being beyond parental control).

there is strong evidence of severe abuse) what recommendations should be made to the court.

1991 saw the implementation of the 1989 Children's Act which provides the framework for all child abuse legislation. Emergency Protection Orders (lasting

TEACHING POINTS

1. Always ask the question, 'Could this injury or symptom be caused by child abuse?'
2. Child abuse can occur with parents from all walks of life.
3. Be aware of the common sorts of injury and how to spot them.
4. Non-specific failure to thrive may be due to child abuse.
5. Referral to hospital is better earlier rather than later in cases of chronic abuse.
6. If a case conference is held it is very important that the general practitioner should present his or her views and take part in any decision-making that occurs.

23 A WHEEZY CHILD

Asthma is one of the most common of all known conditions, affecting about 10% of children. It will therefore count as the most common treatable disorder of childhood, yet there is substantial evidence that it is underdiagnosed and often inadequately treated. Asthma is still responsible for some 2000 deaths each year, is one of the most common causes of school absence and is a frequent limiting factor in a child's sporting activities.

In children, asthma can have a variety of presentations – from the persistently wheezy child to the child with recurrent coughs and colds. It is in this latter group, children with recurrent respiratory symptoms (often with a persistent cough), that the diagnosis is often missed – numerous courses of antibiotics fail to resolve the situation until a bronchodilator is tried, with considerable improvement.

Mrs Spaldwick brought her 4-year-old son, James, to the surgery once again one cold winter morning. 'He's still coughing, doctor,' she said tiredly, 'and he never seems to shake off these colds.' We had seen James with a cough five times in the last 8 months. Each time he had been seen by a different partner and, although one had enquired about a family history of asthma, as yet James had only received cough linctuses or antibiotics. On one occasion a note of a 'slightly wheezy chest' had been made. Today there were again some soft wheezes to be heard in James' chest, but otherwise he was apyrexial with no other signs.

Can a diagnosis of asthma be made?

Yes. Asthma can be defined as 'bronchial hyperreactivity' or 'reversible airways obstruction'. Whatever definition is used, the key to the detection and management of asthma in childhood lies in the recognition of the clinical presentations of asthma in this age group:

1. nocturnal cough
2. persistent cough
3. recurrent 'coughs and colds'
4. exercise-induced cough or dyspnoea
5. wheezing, particularly in response to a respiratory tract infection.

In children, therefore, the important symptom to consider is cough, in particular nocturnal cough. Asthma is the most common cause of a persistent cough in children (other causes being pertussis, chronic respiratory infection, inhaled foreign bodies, cystic fibrosis, hiatus hernia and certain rare anatomical or immune disorders). The child with a nocturnal, persistent or recurrent cough should therefore receive a trial of a bronchodilator. As a further extension of the philosophy, children who wheeze should similarly be assumed to be asthmatic, even if the wheeze is precipitated by a viral respiratory tract infection. Even under the age of 2, where a viral bronchiolitis (caused by respiratory syncytial virus) may cause a wheezy chest, there is evidence to suggest that many of these children have a tendency to wheeze, i.e. asthma. As with persistent cough, there are very few causes of wheezing not attributable to asthma (in children these causes include inhaled foreign bodies, cystic fibrosis, congenital abnormalities and heart disease). In effect, one can say that a child who wheezes usually has asthma.

What would you say to Mrs Spaldwick?

One of the reasons asthma is underdiagnosed is a fear of the word itself. If, as outlined above, one accepts the definition of asthma to include children who wheeze, or whose cough responds to a bronchodilator, then we are talking of a substantial proportion of children on our list (perhaps as many as 10–20% of all children). Since making the diagnosis is the key to giving the correct treatment, the word 'asthma' should not be concealed. The word is, however, a frightening term to the lay public and its introduction into a consultation merits a full explanation of the condition. Mrs Spaldwick should be told that James probably has a mild form of asthma, i.e. his airways tend to narrow when they meet an infection, on exercise or when there is a change in his environment. It should be explained that asthma is a common disorder, affecting about 10% of all children, and there is every expectation (although, of course, no guarantee) that James will 'grow out' of his asthma. Furthermore, Mrs Spaldwick should be reassured that there is a simple treatment to open James' airways and there is no reason why he should not lead as full and active a life as other children.

Are there any questions you would ask Mrs Spaldwick?

It would be appropriate to document James' medical history further by asking the following relevant questions:

- Is there a history of asthma, eczema, hay fever in the family?
- Did James have eczema as a baby?
- Is James' cough mainly nocturnal or does it occur largely during the day?
- Does he cough/wheeze on exercise?
- Are there any pets in the house?
- Does anyone in the family smoke?

As regards further assessment, James is too young to cooperate properly with peak expiratory flow rate measurements, but older children should be able to use a peak flow meter. Similarly, in older children it would be important to have a record of time off school. A blood RAST test would be worth taking in older children to document specific allergies (house dust mite allergy being a particularly important factor in childhood asthma) but blood tests are too invasive for a 4-year-old like James.

How would you approach treatment?

The first step is a full discussion of the principles of treatment with Mrs Spaldwick. She should be given a booklet on asthma and advised on simple measures in the house to reduce the house dust mite. Smoking in the family should be discouraged. A practice nurse is the ideal educator for patients with asthma in the

practice. The British Guidelines are summarized in Box 23.1.

At the age of 4 James could probably just about

Box 23.1 Management of asthma in children under 5 years of age: the British Guidelines

- *Aims*
  Avoidance of provoking factors
  Work towards a self-management plan
  Selection of the best inhaler device
- *Step 1: occasional use of relief bronchodilators*
  Short acting β-agonists (salbutamol is the first line drug of choice) for symptom relief. Mildest cases may respond to oral β-agonists. If inhaled drugs needed more than once a day, move to step 2
- *Step 2: regular inhaled preventer therapy*
  Inhaled short-acting β-agonists as required, *plus*
  Either cromoglycate as powder (20 mg 3–4 times a day) or via a metered dose inhaler and large volume spacer (10 mg t.d.s.), *or* Beclomethasone or budesonide up to 400 µg daily or flucatisone up to 200 µg daily
- *Step 3: increased dose of inhaled steroid*
  Short acting β-agonist as required, *plus* Beclomethasone or budesonide (Pulmicort) increased up to 800 µg or fluticasone (Flixotide) 500 µg daily via large volume spacer. Consider adding a long acting β-agonist or slow-release xanthine
- *Step 4: high-dose inhaled steroids and bronchodilators*
  Inhaled steroids up to 2 mg/day and other treatments as in step 3. Consider adding a long acting β-agonist or slow release xanthines or nebulized β-agonists
- *Stepping down*
  Regularly review the need to step down when indicated. Monitor all changes of treatment clinically by review

Note: Before changing from one step to another check that the treatment is being taken, the inhaler technique is good and the inhaler is appropriate

manage an inhaler with a spacing device (such as a Volumatic or Nebuhaler), rather than relying on an oral syrup. Children under the age of 8 years lack the coordination to use a pressurized inhaler on its own. Whatever system is chosen, the key to success lies in a careful demonstration of the technique of using the system, and time should be spent with Mrs Spaldwick and James to ensure the system chosen is properly used.

The bronchodilator helped James but over the course of the next year he was still subject to occasional attacks of wheeze and nocturnal cough.

What would be the next step?

A good proportion of childhood asthmatics benefit from regular prophylactic therapy. If the only time a child wheezes or coughs is in association with a respiratory tract infection, a bronchodilator alone may suffice. However, if the child is troubled by recurrent cough and wheeze, prophylactic therapy, in the form of sodium cromoglycate or inhaled steroids, is the answer. When using sodium cromoglycates, stress to the mother:

1. Sodium cromoglycate is a preventative treatment, of no use in the acute attack. For an attack of asthma, the bronchodilator should be used.
2. Being preventative, it must be taken regularly, 4 times a day.
3. The benefits of therapy may not be obvious in the first few weeks. The trial of therapy should be for at least 3 months.
4. The aim is for long-term continuous therapy, probably for some years.

With the increasing severity of asthma, sodium cromoglycate may not be sufficient and inhaled steroids may be required. When using inhaled steroids, stress to the mother that:

1. At the dose James is likely to require there will be no stunting of growth.
2. By controlling James's asthma better it will improve his symptoms, exercise tolerance and school attendance (less time off with asthma).
3. They are not the 'dangerous' steroids she may have heard about on the television and they have minimal side-effects when taken by the inhaled route.

James subsequently required inhaled steroids, stabilizing on 50 μg fluticasone twice a day.

TEACHING POINTS

1. Asthma is the most common treatable condition of childhood, affecting about 10% of all children.
2. The clinical presentations of asthma in childhood include nocturnal cough, persistent cough, recurrent 'coughs and colds', exercise-induced cough or dyspnoea and wheezing (particularly in response to a respiratory tract infection).
3. If a child is troubled with recurrent symptoms consider prophylactic therapy with sodium cromoglycate (Intal) or inhaled steroids.
4. There are now well-established guidelines for treatment. British Thoracic Society & National Asthma Campaign. *Thorax* 1997:52 (Suppl 1) S1.

24 A CHILD WITH CROUP

To mothers, croup ranks with convulsions as one of the most worrying of all childhood illnesses. It occurs in very young children, is characterized by a barking cough and noisy stridor and the child looks obviously in distress. Worse still, the symptoms generally develop to their height in the early hours of the morning. Small wonder that croup is a potent cause of many night visits.

To the inexperienced doctor croup seems much less of a problem. However, it is an illness fraught with danger for the newcomer. Croup, by itself, is not always so benign a condition and the airways obstruction can rarely proceed to a dangerous level with serious anoxia requiring tracheal intubation or tracheostomy. Furthermore, it may be difficult to differentiate croup from the more serious, and potentially fatal, epiglottitis. There are few childhood conditions that fill a doctor's heart with terror, but epiglottitis, like meningitis, is one which, once seen, is rarely forgotten. Finally, the parental anxiety aroused by a child with croup can be a fine test of a doctor's ability to calm and reassure patients. It is advisable to be familiar with the diagnosis and management of this fairly common childhood infection.

Carol Todd was an intelligent, but anxious, mother. She lived in a large detached house some 3 miles from the surgery and had two children—Daniel aged 2 and Mark aged 7. She rang at 4 a.m. one winter morning apologetically asking for advice because Daniel had what she thought was croup and she was a little worried because he seemed so distressed and there was nothing she could do to comfort him.

How would you respond to this request?

A request for 'advice' at 4 a.m. cannot always be taken at face value. I had the advantage of knowing Carol very well and her approach to doctors was always apologetic and deferential. This was Carol's way of requesting a visit and I immediately appreciated this.

It may be possible for an experienced general practitioner to give advice on the initial management of croup over the telephone prior to a later visit, providing several conditions are met. The doctor must be thoroughly satisfied it is croup. The croup must be sufficiently mild to be manageable at home and the parents must be capable of coping. Furthermore the doctor must ensure that he or she is kept in touch with progress as, at the earliest indication that there is no improvement with a trial of steam inhalation, a visit is mandatory. It is wise to visit sooner rather than later if the child is under 2 years of age, and another reason for visiting early is to allay parental anxiety—not always easy on the telephone. We would thus recommend an early visit in every case, although it may occasionally be possible to delay a visit for an hour or two in the mildest of cases where steam inhalation hasn't been tried.

With Carol, who had already sat Daniel in a bathroom full of steam, I said I would come and see Daniel as soon as possible and to keep him in the bathroom until I arrived.

What questions might you have asked Carol over the telephone?

I knew Carol and instinctively guessed she was probably right in her diagnosis and management, but must have been very worried. If an unknown patient rings up and requests a visit because a child has 'croup', 'noisy breathing' or a 'bad cough with a bark', questions should be directed at four areas:

1. *General information.* Name, address and age of the child.

2. *Is it croup?* How long had the child been ill? What are his symptoms like—his cough and breathing? Has he a sore throat or fever? Has he had any difficulty with swallowing? Is he dribbling? Is his voice hoarse or muffled? Is he sitting upright or lying down? Is there any possibility of his having inhaled anything?

3. *What is the degree of urgency of the visit?* Is his noisy breathing (stridor) there all the time or is it intermittent? Is it getting worse? Is he restless? Is his colour normal? Is he breathing very quickly? Is his chest heaving in and out?

4. *What have the parents given the child or tried to do to help?* It might be prudent to suggest to the parents over the telephone that they don't try to look in the child's throat (see later). You will be able to assess the degree of anxiety of the parents over the telephone and this in itself may warrant a speedy visit. A doctor who chooses not to visit within a reasonably short time of the request must have a very good reason for his or her decision.

I arrived at Carol's home to find Daniel sitting miserably in the bathroom. His main symptom was a barking cough with a mild and intermittent stridor. He looked reasonably well apart from this, with a normal temperature, good colour and no recession of his chest wall. He was, in fact, quite lively. Carol thought that he had improved in the last hour with the steam but wondered if I could give him anything to calm him down.

What diagnoses might you consider?

Daniel probably had a simple viral croup and was improving with the inhaled steam. The first task must be to exclude the rarer, and more serious, epiglottitis (see Table 24.1). An inhaled foreign body must also be considered in a severe sudden onset of stridor—this is unusual but nevertheless urgent.

Table 24.1 The distinguishing features of croup and epiglottitis

	Croup	Epiglottitis
Age of the child	6 months–3 years	2–4 years
Causative agent	Parainfluenza virus	*Haemophilus influenzae*
Fever	Often none, or mild	>38°C
Length of illness	Often prodromal coryzal symptoms	Rapid course, progressing in hours
Stridor	May be loud	Often muffled, quieter than croup
Sore throat	–	+
Dysphagia, drooling saliva	–	+
Posture		Child prefers sitting upright

Making the diagnosis of croup is not usually too difficult. It affects children from about 6 months to 3 years, being preceded by coryzal symptoms, although these are often mild. The characteristic features are a barking cough, hoarse voice and inspiratory stridor. The child is often afebrile or only slightly febrile.

Acute epiglottitis is a serious infection affecting not just the epiglottis but the whole of the supraglottis. *Haemophilus influenzae* type B is the typical organism in children and is declining because of the HIB vaccination. In adults *Staphylococcus aureus* and *Streptococcus pneumoniae* can also be culprits. Children with bacterial infections are usually very ill, with a temperature, inspiratory and expiratory stridor and frequently dribbling as a result of the swelling.

Affected children are typically 2–4-years-old and become ill with painful dysphagia and stridor within a matter of hours. The stridor helps to distinguish it from the very much more common acute tonsillitis. Urgent referral to hospital is essential and examination inside the mouth should be avoided as it can precipitate respiratory obstruction. Adults are managed in the same way but examining the mouth does not carry the same danger.

How would you assess the severity of the condition and when might you refer a child with croup to the hospital?

Having excluded epiglottitis from your mind, which is a case for very urgent referral to hospital, we must assess the degree of airways obstruction. An impacted inhaled foreign body can cause the most rapid and severe acute obstruction, requiring emergency referral or even tracheotomy in the home. Croup too can occasionally cause severe enough obstruction to merit urgent referral. When faced with a child with croup you should look for five signs, any one of which indicates significant obstruction requiring urgent referral:

1. Cyanosis. An extreme emergency—cardiorespiratory arrest is imminent.
2. General restlessness. Hypoxia causes restlessness, irritability and anxiety. Drowsiness is a grave danger sign when associated with the other symptoms.
3. Rising pulse. A rising tachycardia is a sign of increasing hypoxia but is difficult to measure properly in the excitement of the situation.

4. Intercostal recession, retraction of the sternum during inspiration and supraclavicular recession all indicate severe obstruction, the accessory muscles of respiration doing their best to overcome it.
5. Continuous stridor. Continuous stridor needs an urgent referral before it progresses to complete obstruction and collapse. Stridor with the child peacefully at rest is a particularly ominous sign.

Above all, what is your overall impression of the child? It is best to refer early rather than later and refer if you are at all unhappy with the child. Remember the five signs and pay particular attention to the colour of the child, the degree of restlessness, dyspnoea, significant chest wall retraction and whether the stridor is continuous and present at rest. It is only with experience of seeing many children with croup that you will be able to form a really good impression of the severity of a given case but these signs form an invaluable guide.

Is there any treatment to offer Daniel?

Traditional treatment has been sitting the child in a bathroom full of steam. There is now evidence for the value of steroids in treating acute croup. The current treatment of choice for moderate/severe croup is budesonide using a nebulizer. Budesonide is available as Respules, which are single dose units for nebulization containing 250 or 500 µg/ml (dose for croup is 2 mg nebulized as a single dose or 2×1 mg doses 30 minutes apart). While budesonide helps in the acute stage, the child may still need hospital admission. Many general practitioners carry a nebulizer for emergency use and croup is another condition that can now be treated by nebulized therapy. The question of other drug therapy rarely arises—sedatives are, of course, contraindicated. If you decide to manage a child with croup at home, monitor progress closely.

It is hoped that you will never be faced with the management of that most extreme of all emergencies, a complete airways obstruction with the imminent danger of arrest. The time-honoured size 14 Medicut inserted between the thyroid and cricoid cartilages anteriorly in the midline may then save a life. All doctors should carry a size 14 Medicut in their emergency bags.

Daniel was already improving by the time I arrived. Carol must be told that if she is unhappy, the stridor gets worse and Daniel more restless, she should call you again, but in any case you will visit before morning surgery. Explain to Carol that sedatives, cough mixtures and antibiotics are unlikely to benefit Daniel and may obscure how well he is doing.

I visited at 8 a.m. the next morning and Daniel was much improved. He still had a cough but was coughing much less frequently and had virtually no residual stridor. I managed a much needed cup of tea with Carol before morning surgery.

TEACHING POINTS

1. Be wary of a diagnosis of 'croup'.
2. Distinguish croup from epiglottitis and inhalation of a foreign body.
3. Know when to refer to hospital.
4. Children affected with epiglottitis are typically 2–4 years of age and present with painful dysphagia and stridor in a matter of hours. Urgent referral is needed.

As immunization programmes become widespread, the general practitioner becomes less familiar with the presentations of the common infectious diseases.

In fact 'Immunization programmes are the most evidence-based and cost-effective procedures carried out in primary care' (Grob *RCGP Members Book* 1996 p. 102). Communicating quality information to parents and involving them in the immunization programme is an antidote to the premature release in the press of reports of alarming side-effects and rare complications before they have been properly evaluated and published in peer review journals.

Every now and then an atypical case will arise or a parent ask a searching question. It is well worthwhile outlining the course of an infectious illness to a parent as this may save several consultations for the same illness. Some knowledge of the incubation periods and the infectivity of the common infectious illnesses is required, as there will be many occasions on which your advice will be sought with regard to a child going to school and what to do about his younger sister. Common infectious illnesses are listed in Table 25.1.

In the United Kingdom certain common infectious diseases are notifiable. These are shown in Box 25.1. Other common infectious diseases are not notifiable, e.g. chickenpox. Immunization is very much part of a general practice; in our practice immunization of young children is carried out on the premises in a special clinic. Increasingly, computer-linked systems ensure that all children are called for immunization at the correct time. The introduction of the target payment system for immunization has added a new impetus to achieve high rates for immunization uptake. Over 90% of Health Authorities have achieved about 95% coverage of their populations in most primary vaccination courses.

Box 25.1 List of notifiable diseases

- Anthrax
- Cholera
- Diphtheria
- Hepatitis A
- Hepatitis B
- Hepatitis C
- Measles
- Meningitis, Haemophilus and meningococcal ABC
- Mumps
- Pertussis
- Pneumococcal infections, e.g. pneumonia
- Polio
- Rabies
- Rubella
- Smallpox
- Tetanus
- Tuberculosis
- Typhoid
- Varicella notifiable in Scotland and Northern Ireland
- Yellow fever

Table 25.1 Common infectious illnesses

	Incubation period (days)	Period of infectivity
Measles (less common today than previously)	8–15	From prodromal symptoms to 5 days after onset of rash
Rubella (German measles)	14–21 (usually 14–15)	From 7 days before rash to 5 days after
Chickenpox	11–21 (usually 14–15)	From 2 days before rash until 7 days after last crop
Mumps	12–28	From 3 days before swelling until 7 days after subsidence of swelling
Whooping cough	7–10	From 2 days before symptoms up to 5 weeks after start of a cough

Mrs Wilson makes an appointment to see you about the MMR vaccine, having recently read of a possible association with inflammatory bowel disease. She asks, 'Should my baby have MMR as his father has Crohn's disease?'

Until recently the answer would have been a simple 'Yes' but the National Association for Crohn's disease and Colitis have produced an information leaflet which refers to research suggesting a link between MMR vaccine and the presence of Crohn's lesion. It states that the measles virus is one of the possible triggers, based on a Swedish paper which suggests that at times of measles epidemics children exposed to the measles virus seem to have more likelihood of developing Crohn's disease. Another study identified measles virus particles in areas of bowel which have been damaged with Crohn's disease. The vaccine used in MMR is a weaker form of the virus and raises the possibility that this may be causing the disease. Rightly, the article goes on to say that cause and effect have not been established and that more research is needed; the possibility not the probability exists at present. It says that the vaccination policy is a sensible one. On balance, MMR vaccination benefits still outweigh the risks and should be encouraged.

This is the wording of a poster we used in the surgery waiting room:

- The MMR jab is very safe.
- It is good at preventing measles, mumps and German measles—all illnesses which can cause serious problems and so are worth being protected against.
- There is no evidence of a link between the MMR jab and Crohn's disease or autism.
- There is no need for each part of the MMR to be given separately. It may even be more risky to do so.
- We strongly believe children should be given the MMR jab at the recommended times.

When should a child be immunized against measles, and are there any contraindications to immunization?

In the United Kingdom the MMR vaccine (measles, mumps, rubella—a live vaccine) is advised for all children near the beginning of the second year of life; between 12 and 15 months. If given too early, i.e. under 12 months, there is poorer antibody formation due to the presence of antibodies from the mother.

The morbidity associated with measles justifies its prevention. Parents should be warned that some children develop a transient febrile illness with a rash about 8 days following immunization and rarely a parotid swelling will appear about the third week. Children are not infectious post vaccination. MMR vaccine may also be used for prophylaxis if given within 72 hours of exposure to the measles virus.

Contraindications to MMR vaccine include:

1. General contraindications to all live vaccines, viz:
   - Pregnancy (but hardly applicable here!)
   - Acute febrile illness (not just snuffles)
   - Patients immunosuppressed by treatment or with hypogamma-globulinaemia
   - Patients on steroids
   - Patients with malignant conditions
   - Radiotherapy given to patients
   - Within 3 weeks of another live vaccine being given. If it is necessary to give more than one live vaccine at the same time, they should be given simultaneously in different sites (unless a combined preparation is used) or separated by a period of at least 3 weeks.

2. In addition there are more specific contra-indications:
   - Active tuberculosis
   - Hypersensitivity to egg protein or neomycin. Note that egg allergy must be of an anaphylactoid nature (urticaria, breathing difficulties, etc.) for this to be a contraindication
   - Blood dyscrasias, e.g. thrombocytopenia
   - Within 3 weeks of an immunoglobulin injection

3. Note that convulsions in the patient or family are no longer a contraindication—but advice should be given to the mother on how to reduce the temperature. Note also that a history of measles, mumps or rubella is no contraindication to vaccination. Children with no record of MMR vaccination should receive a dose at 4–5 years old before beginning school. If for any reason MMR vaccine is given to postpubertal females remember to advise against pregnancy for 3 months post vaccination.

IMMUNIZATION

It is important to be familiar with the standard schedule for immunization (Table 25.2).

1. DPT (diphtheria/pertussis/tetanus)

The triple vaccine is given by intramuscular injection. The main controversy lies with the pertussis component. The 1981 report of the National Childhood Encephalopathy Study indicates that the risk of persisting neurological damage from the vaccine is 1 in 310 000; this is a much smaller risk of damage than the incidence of death from whooping cough, which is estimated at 1 in 3000.

PERTUSSIS

What is it?

Pertussis is a highly infectious bacterial disease caused by *Bordetella pertussis* spread by droplet infection; incubation 7–10 days. The onset is insidious with a catarrhal stage followed by an irritating cough that becomes paroxysmal. It often lasts 2–3 months. The typical indrawing of breath and the accompanying stridor, once heard, will not be forgotten. I find a demonstration to the parents of the difference between paroxysmal cough and a repetitive choking cough often clarifies their description. I have also diagnosed pertussis from a tape recording of the sufferer taken during paroxysms at home. Early diagnosis is important because erythromycin is effective in the early stages.

The story of immunization is a salutory one. Before immunization was introduced in the 1950s, annual notifications exceeded 100 000. Following its introduction in 1972, when acceptance was 80%, there were only 2069 notifications. Because there was public anxiety over the safety and efficacy of the vaccine following some very poor quality public debate, including the promotion of a homeopathic alternative, acceptance rates fell to 30% and major epidemics followed, with 100 000 notifications in 1977–1979 and 1981–1983. Public confidence slowly returned and in 1986 an epidemic was cut short. By 1992 the uptake had risen to 92%. By 1995 coverage was 94% and there were 1873 notifications, the lowest level since records began.

It is recommended that the vaccine be given to all children from the age of 2 months unless there is a genuine contraindication (Box 25.2).

The acellular vaccine is incorporated in a number of vaccination programmes abroad.

Table 25.2 Immunization schedule

Vaccine	Age		Notes
D/T/P and Hib Polio	1st dose 2nd dose 3rd dose	2 months 3 months 4 months	Primary Course
Measles/mumps/rubella (MMR)	12–15 months		Can be given at any age over 12 months
Booster DT and polio, MMR second dose	3–5 years		Three years after completion of primary course
BCG	10–14 years or infancy		
Booster tetanus diphtheria and polio	13–18 years		

Children should therefore have received the following vaccines:
By 6 months: 3 doses of DTP, Hib and polio
By 15 months: Measles/mumps/rubella
By school entry: 4th DT and polio; second dose measles/mumps/rubella
Between 10 and 14 years: BCG
Before leaving school: 5th polio and tetanus diphtheria (Td).

Box 25.2 Contraindications to whooping cough vaccination

1. Contraindicated in children who have: history of any severe local or general reaction to a preceding dose
2. Postpone in children who have any acute illness. (Minor infections without fever or systemic upset do not count)
3. The following are not so much contraindications as points deserving consideration when deciding whether or not to give the vaccine. In these cases discuss with a paediatrician:
   a. Children who have previously had a convulsion or apnoeic attack
   b. Children with a history of brain damage in the neonatal period
   c. Children with first-degree relatives (parents or siblings) with epilepsy

2. Polio

A live vaccine containing all three types of polio virus and given orally. As well as general contraindications to live vaccines, remember diarrhoea and vomiting and also sensitivity to penicillin, neomycin, streptomycin and polymyxin (although the sensitivity must be of a truly anaphylactoid nature, considering the minimal traces present).

3. BCG

This is an attenuated strain of bacillus and is given to school children who are tuberculin negative. It is also given at birth to infants of families with a history of active tuberculosis; in Leicester it is given to all babies of Asian mothers.

4. Hib vaccine

Hib stands for *Haemophilus influenzae* type b vaccine. It can cause meningitis, epiglottitis and septicaemia; rarely causes septic arthritis, osteomyelitis, cellulitis, pneumonia and pericarditis. Hib immunization has successfully reduced the incidence of Hib from 627 in 1992 to 39 in 1995. Hib vaccine is not live. The primary course is of 3 doses, with an interval of a month between each dose. Hib vaccine can be mixed with DTP vaccine for simultaneous administration (i.e. in the form of a single injection. Adverse reactions include swelling and redness at the local injection site.

Contraindications to Hib vaccination are acute illness (postpone the vaccination) and a previous reaction to the vaccine.

The general practitioner is not likely to meet many complications of vaccination, but because of the rare occurrence of anaphylactic shock some adrenaline for injection should always be at hand.

In setting up an immunization clinic one of the main problems is to ensure that everyone is aware of the contraindications. In this context a simple written card can be compiled (as in Box 25.3) to be read by all those presenting for immunization; the vast majority being mothers bringing their children to the clinic.

The consent of the mother should be obtained, preferably as a written record before each procedure, after the child's fitness and suitability have been established. As regards the site of injection, the current guidelines are that for subcutaneous or intramuscular injections the anterolateral aspect of the thigh or the upper arm are recommended. In the buttock, the upper outer quadrant should be used. There is still a vigorous debate over the best site for injection.

Box 25.3 lists the questions that patients should be asked.

Box 25.3 Questions for patients—all immunizations and vaccinations—to be answered by, or on behalf of, the person who is to be immunized

1. Have you or any member of your family a history of:
   Fits?
   Seizures?
   Epilepsy?
   Convulsions?
   Brain damage?
2. Do you suffer from:
   Hodgkin's disease?
   Leukaemia?
   Lymphoma?
   Have you received radiotherapy or chemotherapy?
3. Have you any chronic serious illness, e.g. bronchitis or heart disease, asthma or eczema?
4. Are you pregnant?
5. Have you any present illness, e.g. respiratory illness, diarrhoea or sickness?
6. Have you had any trouble with previous injections?
7. Are you sensitive to:
   Penicillin?
   Neomycin?
   Streptomycin?
   Polymyxin?
   Eggs?
   Rabbits?
8. Have the members of your household not had their full course of polio injections?
9. Have you had any injection within the last 3 weeks?

If the answer to any of these questions is 'yes', or if you have any problems, please inform the nurse or doctor before having the injection.

CHICKENPOX

Chickenpox is not a difficult disease to diagnose. My 10-year-old patient, Sandra Church, had been feeling mildly ill for about 2 days and now some itchy spots had appeared on her trunk. She had a mild temperature of 37.6°C. Her mother asked me if she could have a steroid cream to relieve the itching of the rash as it had helped her sister's eczema. I advised against steroid cream and recommended the application of calamine lotion.

The clinical features and complications (there are few in childhood) of chickenpox are portrayed in Figure 25.1. There are few prodromal signs and this stage is very short, the rash appearing usually within a day of the illness.

Mrs Church was not sure if she had had chickenpox as a child. Can adults get it, she asked?

One attack of chickenpox usually confers permanent immunity and about three-quarters of adults have had chickenpox. However, it can and does occur in adults, when the rash may be worse and constitutional symptoms more severe. There is no specific treatment in the uncomplicated case.

What is the relationship between chickenpox and shingles?

The varicella-zoster virus seems to cause both. The theory is that the virus remains in the dorsal root ganglia to be reactivated in later life and cause shingles. There are three interesting points to ponder:

1. Patients with herpes zoster (shingles) can trans-

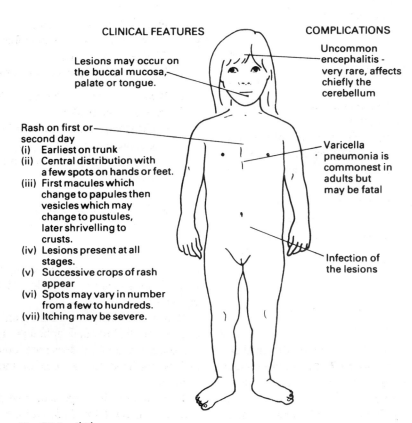

CLINICAL FEATURES

Lesions may occur on the buccal mucosa, palate or tongue.

Rash on first or second day
(i) Earliest on trunk
(ii) Central distribution with a few spots on hands or feet.
(iii) First macules which change to papules then vesicles which may change to pustules, later shrivelling to crusts.
(iv) Lesions present at all stages.
(v) Successive crops of rash appear
(vi) Spots may vary in number from a few to hundreds.
(vii) Itching may be severe.

COMPLICATIONS

Uncommon encephalitis - very rare, affects chiefly the cerebellum

Varicella pneumonia is commonest in adults but may be fatal

Infection of the lesions

Fig. 25.1 Chickenpox.

mit chickenpox. Thus a child taken to visit granny with shingles may, 11–21 days later, develop chickenpox.

2. Patients developing zoster are usually elderly but can be young. There is usually a previous history of chickenpox, but there are cases where a primary infection with varicella-zoster seems to produce shingles rather than chickenpox.

3. Chickenpox and herpes zoster have occasionally been recorded in the same person.

Are there any treatments active against the chickenpox virus?

Yes. Aciclovir given shortly after the onset of chickenpox will attenuate the illness. It can be given orally or intravenously. Adults (often more severely affected) are worth treating, as are the immuno-suppressed, children with severe attacks, those with heart/lung disorders, those with complications and those with significant skin diseases (including eczema). Note that a pregnant woman in contact with chickenpox needs an antibody test and, if not immune, should be given varicella-zoster immunoglobulin.

MENINGITIS

The publicity about meningitis has presented general practitioners with a difficult problem.

A call is received from a parent, aware of this condition, whose child has become pyrexial and is seeking help, often in a covert manner, e.g. 'I should like some advice…'

It is helpful to the doctor if the fear of meningitis is made explicit but in any case you should be prepared to make an initial assessment. The most important thing is to be aware of the possibility. The diagnosis is summarized in Box 25.4.

What history would you record and what examination would you make?

Generally does the child look well or ill? Is there a pyrexia? Is he or she rousable? Is feeding normal? Has there been vomiting or diarrhoea? Is there a rash? Is the kernig test positive?

It can be quite difficult to elicit neck rigidity. Can you bend the child's neck forward in the lying

---

Box 25.4 Diagnosis of meningitis

- Classical features: headache, neck/back stiffness, nausea and vomiting and photophobia with fever and drowsiness
- Convulsions may be a feature in infants and young children but neck and back stiffness are rare. Flaccidity is much more common
- In meningococcal infections diarrhoea is sometimes an important non-specific symptom and a petechial rash is the warning sign of urgency
- Kernig's sign may be present and the child may not be able to touch the chin on the chest (a tip for performing this test is to ask the child to kiss a knee)
- A bulging fontanelle in neonates should be sought.

- *Symptoms of meningitis*
  Headache
  Fever
  Vomiting
  Neck stiffness/joint pains
  Drowsiness or confusion/coma
  Dislike of bright lights
  Rash of red purple spots or bruises

- *What to look for in babies with meningitis*
  Pale or blotchy skin
  Child is unresponsive or hard to wake
  High-pitched or moaning cry
  Rash of red/purple spots or bruises
  Fretfulness
  Fever
  Refusing feeds or vomiting

---

position? Many children, especially if frightened, can resist this manoeuvre. As in Box 25.4, see if the child can kiss the knees.

Rarely tonsillitis can cause pain in the neck that can be confusing, and although this referred pain can seem suspicious it does not produce neck stiffness and is confined to the area of the fourth cervical vertebra.

If meningitis is suspected, emergency antibiotics should be given (Box 25.5) and the child transported urgently to hospital.

Box 25.5 Emergency treatment for suspected meningitis

1. Administer intravenous or intramuscular antibiotic benzyl penicillin to all patients (unless previous anaphylaxis) Cefotaxime when penicillin cannot be given
2. Admit to hospital, transport with oxygen if comatosed or shocked

Dosage

Benzylpenicillin	1200 mg for over 10-year-olds
	600 mg for 1–10-year-olds
	300 mg for under 1-year-olds
Cefotaxime	2000 mg for over 10-year-olds
	See literature for doses for under 10 years old

Prevention
Soon it is proposed to introduce a vaccine

INFLUENZA AND PNEUMONIA

Influenza is an acute viral infection of the respiratory tract affecting all age groups and characterized by an abrupt onset of fever, shivering, headache, myalgia, and sometimes prostration. A dry cough is very common and often there is a sore throat. It is a self-limiting disease: recovery in 2–7 days. Complications are bronchitis, bacterial pneumonia and otitis media (in children). The incubation period is 1–3 days.

Although the mortality rate is low, most deaths occur in those with underlying conditions, particularly respiratory and cardiac. Primary influenzal pneumo-nia is rare but has a high death rate. It is a disease that occurs in very variable numbers, at time reaching epidemic proportions. Even in a quiet year 3000–4000 deaths may be attributed to influenza. In an epidemic year, such as 1989–1990, this figure rose to 30 000.

Pneumococcal pneumonia is the fourth biggest killer in the UK. One in 1000 adults contract this infection each year and there is a mortality of 20%. The pneumococcus is also one of the most common causes of bacteraemia and meningitis. About 9000 people are expected to die from this infection each year.

It is for these reasons that, as a practice, we offer an influenza immunization to all our elderly patients, patients with cardiovascular and respiratory disease, those without a spleen, diabetics, those with chronic renal and liver problems or who are immune deficient, and pneumococcal vaccination to those among them who have not already had it. (Note there are special contraindications to pneumococcal vaccine—consult a formulary guide first).

TEACHING POINTS

1. Revise the immunization schedule and the contraindications to vaccination.
2. MMR vaccine is a live vaccine given near the beginning of the second year of life.
3. Chickenpox is easy to diagnose, has a usual incubation period of about 14–15 days, and has few complications in childhood.
4. Beware meningitis!
5. Revise the indications for influenza and penumococcal vaccination.

26 HEADACHES

Headaches are a very common experience. Ninety per cent of the population will have had this symptom within 1 year and 20% will have had a headache within 2 weeks. It is the tenth most common presenting symptom in general practice. That there are usually no serious underlying causes is commonly recognized by both doctor and patient, but the patient expects reassurance and symptomatic relief. One-fifth of those attending neurological outpatients' clinics complain of headache.

The diagnosis of migraine is made on the history of:

- an episodic throbbing headache lasting 4–72 hours
- the headache is usually unilateral
- in 70% of cases the headache is associated with nausea/vomiting.

Only about a fifth of patients have neurological symptoms in the form of an aura preceding the headache. These symptoms may be visual (fortification spectra, blurred vision, teichopsia), sensory (paraesthesiae, numbness) or speech disturbances.

The vicar's wife, Mrs Ruth Cramphorn, 50-years-old, comes in complaining somewhat breathlessly of headache.

What questions would you ask her?

You should try to obtain a clear account of the symptoms to elicit the site of the headache. Is it unilateral, occipital or frontal? The quality and nature of the pain—is it a tight band or a dull ache? Is it burning or throbbing? Its intensity. The more florid the adjectives used to describe it the more likely is the headache to be associated with psychological stress. Its duration—has it been present for less than 48 hours? Does it come and go? If so how often and at what time of the day? Have there been any associated symptoms, for example vomiting, nausea, flashing lights (teichopsia)? Are there secondary features, such as signs of

respiratory tract infection? It is important to know whether or not she is on any current treatment and what, if anything, she has done to relieve the present symptoms. She should also be asked her views on the condition.

The diagnosis in the majority of headaches will depend on the history, and the physical examination will usually be negative.

What, then, are the cardinal features of a headache? Table 26.1 shows the conditions which can present with headache, and are arranged in the order of frequency with which they are likely to occur. In general practice careful questioning about past experiences of a similar headache, its nature, site, and association with aura, teichopsia, nausea and/or vomiting, should largely distinguish the so-called migraines and tension headaches from other causes of headaches. The time scales are particularly helpful because migraine is normally a headache of recent onset associated with nausea and vomiting and is usually unilateral. There is frequently a past and family history (in 70% of patients).

Headaches of more than 48 hours' duration which

Table 26.1 Relative probabilities for possible causes of headache per 1000 population in a year

Cause	Probability
Respiratory disease	400
Anxiety	38
Depression	36
Migraine	8
Cervical spondylosis	7
Cerebrovascular accident	6
Headache—non-specific	4
Sinusitis	2
Refractive errors	0.7
Malignant hypertension	0.4
Meningitis	0.2
Meningococcal meningitis	0.1
Brain tumour	0.1

are different from the patient's previous experience should arouse suspicion.

In this case she describes a pain in the occipital region which feels like a tight band and which radiates down her neck.

What examination should you make?

Inspection

She appeared a healthy, plump, slightly anxious woman whose attempts at weight control had succumbed to the temptations of the Women's Institute Saturday teas.

Palpation

There are no tender spots on the temporal arteries or the scalp and the cervical muscle appears tense.

Movement of the neck is normal with a slight limitation of forward flexion.

You take her blood pressure, not because it is a common cause of headache, but you notice that it has not been recorded before and you know that she may have some expectations that you will do this.

Her temperature is normal and so is the appearance of her optic fundi.

What should you do next?

The picture emerging is one of a tension headache and Mrs Cramphorn's demeanour and appearance support this view. It is always helpful to know what has brought about the present consultation and what the patient thinks about her symptoms.

The reasons why patients consult about symptoms are many, but can usually be categorized into one of the following groups:

1. a new symptom
2. a symptom which has persisted longer than usual, or is more severe
3. a symptom which presents a threat to either the social or work commitments
4. similarity of a symptom to that of another person for whom it has had serious implications
5. a symptom which, when discussed with family or friends, occasioned the advice to consult a doctor
6. failure of own diagnosis.

You ask her what brought her to see you on this occasion, and she says that she has been very busy recently. She has been nursing an aunt who had a cerebral haemorrhage which developed after a sudden and disabling headache. She is also very involved in the local amateur dramatic production and is about to attend the dress rehearsal on the following day.

This information allows you to make a tentative diagnosis of tension headache associated with a recent unpleasant experience and increasing commitments. You can reassure her that there is no evidence that she is likely to have a stroke, and as her aunt was not a blood relative there is no hereditary risk. She is also under significant pressure and experiencing a headache from tension in her neck muscles. (A vestigial form of the startle reflex in animals.) You advise that she should ask her sister to help with the aunt until the play is over and you offer her some analgesia to tide her over the current period.

MIGRAINE

This case was a tension headache. The management of migraine is also a very common problem. Let us look more closely at some of the difficulties. Box 26.1 summarizes some migraine statistics.

Box 26.1 Migraine: some statistics

- One in five persons suffers from migraine
- 4% of men and 8% of women present to their general practitioner with migraine for the first time
- 30% of patients have at least one attack a month
- 10% of sufferers are severely incapacitated
- 30% of sufferers are moderately incapacitated
- 60% of sufferers are mildly incapacitated
- Of women suffering from migraine, 46% have never consulted their doctor
- 12% of all general practitioner consultations have headache as one symptom

Management of migraine

1. Reassurance, but not too readily with insufficient examination or explanation.

2. Advice: simple procedures if not already tried; a cold compress, lying in a darkened room, aspirin or paracetamol. Try to identify a precipitating factor from the list given in Box 26.2. Take treatment in anticipation of an early attack—trigger factors can be used to predict vulnerable times.

3. For mild attacks of migraine, paracetamol or aspirin may suffice, or combinations of paracetamol and codeine. In acute attacks nausea and vomiting may be a problem necessitating the use of antiemetics like metoclopramide or prochlorperazine (Fig. 26.1).

Box 26.2 Migraine: a list of trigger factors

Anxiety	Fasting	Change of
Anger	Dieting	climate
Worry	Irregular meals	Bright sunlight
Depression	Toothache	Artificial light
Shock	Tender skin	Glare
Excitement	Chocolate	Flickering TV
Overexertion	Cheese	Loud noise
Bending	Fried food	Intense smells
Stooping	Citrus fruits	Smoking
Changing job	Red wine	Very hot baths
Holiday	Menstruation	Sleeping
Shift work	The pill	tablets
Travel	The menopause	High blood
Late rising		pressure

Buccastem is a useful preparation of prochlorperazine for migraine, being a tablet placed between the upper lips and gums and left to dissolve. Non-steroidal anti-inflammatories are worth a try but clearly not if nausea/vomiting are prominent features.

4. If these fail use a $5HT_1$ agonist (Table 26.2). Their advantages are:

-   a >70% success rate in relieving the acute attack
-   can be given at any stage during an attack (but best given early)
-   they relieve the associated symptoms of nausea/vomiting as well as the headache.

The $5HT_1$ agonists have now replaced ergotamine preparations, which are obsolete.

Contraindications include uncontrolled hypertension and ischaemic heart disease; check for possible drug interactions before use.

Prophylaxis

For patients who suffer more than two disabling attacks per month or who have frequent major attacks unresponsive to acute therapy, some form of prophylaxis should be considered. The main choices are given

---

Table 26.2 $5HT_1$ agonists available

Drug	Form
Naratriptan	Tablet
Rizatriptan	Tablet, lyophilisate
Sumatriptan	Tablet, nasal spray, injection
Zolmitriptan	Tablet

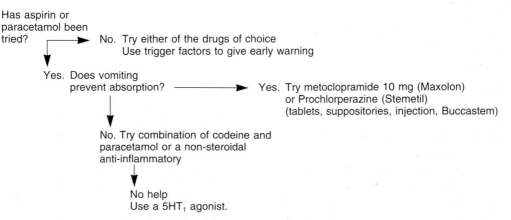

Fig. 26.1 Management of migraine: the acute attack

Box 26.3 Choice of prophylaxis for migraine

1. Beta-blockers, e.g. propranolol 80–160 mg daily
2. Pizotifen (Sanomigran), e.g. 1.5 mg nocte
3. Regular naproxen (Synflex, Naprosyn)
4. Low dose amitriptyline, e.g. 25 mg nocte
5. Regular aspirin
6. For hospital use only, methysergide (Deseril)—can be effective but there is a risk of retroperitoneal fibrosis

in Box 26.3. You need weeks to assess the benefit of prophylaxis and prophylaxis should be prescribed for 6–12 months before trying to withdraw the drug.

TEACHING POINTS

1. Headaches are an extremely common experience.
2. A careful history is essential; it is often all you have to go on.
3. Always find out why this patient consults you now. It will give the diagnosis in most cases.
4. Consider prophylaxis for some patients.

27 A VAGUE PRESENTATION: JAUNDICE

From time to time patients present with vague symptoms which defy categorization—stories of feeling unwell, tiredness, not feeling right, and so forth. Faced with such a challenge a doctor has no alternative but to resort to basic techniques of history-taking and examination, going systematically through the possibilities in order either to eliminate or to uncover the more obscure conditions. Fortunately time is on our side and it is not necessary to make a complete diagnosis at the first encounter. Usually a number of possibilities must be considered and a few basic screening tests performed. A further consultation at a later date is important to review the situation.

Such a case was a 25-year-old housewife, Mrs Hilary Crane-Ley, with two children, who presented complaining of feeling unwell. She had been discharged from hospital following a tonsillectomy 2 weeks previously. Close questioning revealed that she just did not feel well. She was tired and off her food but both these symptoms were attributable to the recent operation.

On examination she was apyrexial with a slough on the tonsillar fauces. She did not look particularly ill.

What possibilities do you consider?

Box 27.1 summarizes the main possibilities.

In all vague presentations the picture is never as barren as it appears in examples. The patient, his or her appearance and disposition, the way the story is told, all supply a wealth of clues which are difficult to capture in the written word.

What impression has the patient made on you? Take the most obvious things first.

This patient is a non-attender, she has just had an operation, proceed from there.

Box 27.1 Some of the more important causes of tiredness

1. Depression/anxiety. Psychological problems are the most common cause
2. Secondary infection, either local or systemic. Major sites are urine or chest
3. Anaemia
4. Subacute bacterial endocarditis
5. Too early mobilization
6. Drugs or smoking
7. Alcohol
8. Hypothyroidism
9. Diabetes mellitus
10. Connective tissue disorders
11. Undiagnosed neoplasms

What questions would you ask that would help to clarify the picture?

First of all the timing of feeling ill. Whether it preceded the operation or only came on afterwards; how long she had been feeling like that; whether it was of sudden onset or gradual onset, and what she particularly notices and how it affects her. General questions about her sleep pattern, the presence or absence of a cough, whether she smokes, her appetite, questions about shortness of breath, and whether she is taking any tablets (e.g. oral contraceptives), her bowel action, micturition, and whether she has any pain in her legs. Questions of a more general nature asked in an open-ended way are more helpful than when a specific condition is being sought.

Unfortunately the answers to these are of little help and you learn no more than is available already. You decide to perform a urine examination and a full blood count and ask her to return in a week's time. At this stage no diagnosis has been made.

Boxes 27.2 to 27.7 summarize some of the information

Box 27.2 The significance of urine microscopy

Casts due to coagulation of protein in tubules
Epithelial casts + RBCs = acute nephritis
Epithelial casts + granular casts
      = inflammation and
       degeneration of tubules
Hyaline casts occur in small numbers in normal
  urine
Hyaline casts in excess = chronic nephritis

Box 27.3 Cause of sterile pyuria

1. Renal TB
2. Analgesic nephropathy
3. Renal calculi
4. Drugs—analgesics
     diuretics
     Jectofer
5. Non-specific urethritis

Box 27.4 Causes of albuminuria

1. Febrile illness
2. Toxaemia of pregnancy
3. Orthostatic albuminuria
4. Glomerulonephritis
5. Tubal necrosis
6. Pyelonephritis
7. Nephrotic syndrome
8. Congestive cardiac failure
9. Multiple myeloma
10. Drugs
11. Nephrocalcinosis

Box 27.5 Drugs which may cause albuminuria

1. Penicillin   } either by hypersensitivity
2. Sulphonamides } or by crystallization
3. Tetracycline
4. Analgesics
5. Vitamin D overdose
6. Mercurials
7. Penicillamine
8. Troxidone

Box 27.6 Blood: causes of hypochromic anaemia

1. Iron deficiency
2. Infection
3. Rheumatoid arthritis } usually
4. Malignancy   } normochromic
5. Thalassaemia
6. Sideroblastic anaemia

Box 27.7 Blood: causes of megaloblastic anaemia

1. Folate deficiency	*Anti-folate drugs* Methotrexate Cholestyramine Anticonvulsants Ethanol Oral contraceptives

2. Vitamin B_{12} deficiency	a. Intrinsic factor deficiency
	b. Post-gastrectomy
	c. Malabsorption
	d. Inadequate diet
	e. Drugs: PAS
	     Colchicine
	     Neomycin
	     Metformin

that might be obtained from examination of the urine or blood.

Mrs Crane-Ley comes back to the surgery saying that she feels very much worse, and you notice now that her skin has a distinct lemon-coloured tinge. Her conjunctivae are yellow. On further questioning, she says that her urine has become dark and her stools are pale. She is not complaining of any itch.

 On examination she is now clearly jaundiced with a tender palpable liver one finger's breadth below the right costal margin. She also has minimal palmar erythema but no other abnormal signs. The blood report is not available.

What possibilities do you now consider?

The most common form of jaundice seen in general practice in younger patients is hepatitis A but other possibilities must be considered.

Did she have an injection 3 months previously? This might suggest that she has developed hepatitis B. Has she got glandular fever, or other conditions which can have jaundice as a complication? Could she have gallstones? Could her jaundice have been precipitated by an anaesthetic? Did she have a blood transfusion? Could this be halothane jaundice or from other drugs? The possibilities seem endless.

How does one start narrowing the field?

It is unlikely that anyone faced with jaundice in a patient like this and who considers the difficulties of diagnosis would not refer to a book for guidance. Table 27.1 and Boxes 27.8 and 27.9 indicate the main possibilities. With careful consideration we can eliminate much:

1. The jaundice appears obstructive. She has pale stools and dark urine.
2. There is a palpable tender liver.
3. On questioning, she did not have any injections 3 months ago and knows of no one who has had jaundice.
4. She is a non-smoker and non-drinker, and is not taking any drugs except the oral contraceptives which she has been on for 4 years. She did not have a blood transfusion.

The probabilities, then, narrow, and hepatitis A would appear top of the list. Halothane jaundice occurs mainly after repeated anaesthetics and is usually of sudden onset and rapidly progressive. Oral contraceptives remain a possibility but usually cause a subclinical jaundice.

Table 27.1 Classification of jaundice

Type	Cause
Prehepatic	Haemolysis
	Gilbert's syndrome
Hepatic	Hepatitis: viral
	drug
	alcohol
	Cirrhosis
	Sex hormones
Cholestatic	Cancer of bile ducts
	Gallstones
	Cancer of head of pancreas

Box 27.8   The causes of hepatomegaly

1. Raised venous pressure	Congestive cardiac failure
2. Degenerative	Fatty infiltration Early cirrhosis
3. Neoplastic	Primary or secondary Lymphoma
4. Infective	a. Viral: infectious hepatitis infectious mononucleosis
	b. Bacterial: TB brucellosis
	c. Protozoal: malaria amoebic, toxoplasmosis
	d. Parasitic: hydatid cyst
5. Storage disorders	
6. Biliary obstruction	
7. Congenital	Polycystic disease

Box 27.9   Some drugs causing jaundice

• Anaesthetics	Halothane
• Antihypertensives	Methyldopa
• Psychotropic	Chlorpromazine
	Phenothiazines
	Amitriptyline
	Benzodiazepines
• Anti-inflammatory	Phenylbutazone
	Oxyphenbutazone
	Indomethacin
• Antituberculous	PAS
	Rifampicin
	Ethambutol
• Antibiotics	Erythromycin
	Tetracycline
	Ampicillin
	Sulphonamides
	Nitrofurantoin
• Antidiabetic	Chlorpropamide
	Tolbutamide
• Cytotoxic	Methotrexate

Liver function tests are likely to show an obstructive pattern. There is the problem in taking a suitable specimen to be handled by laboratory staff. The rules for taking this specimen are as follows:

1. Gloves should be worn while obtaining the intravenous sample.
2. The specimens should be separately labelled and should be sealed in a polythene bag.
3. The laboratory request form should be marked 'Undiagnosed Jaundice'.
4. It is then tested for viral hepatitis before proceeding to other liver function tests (Table 27.2).

What should the patient be told and how would you manage her now?

The jaundice occurred without any other associated events. Most cases in general practice can be attributed to hepatitis A and are managed mainly without referral. If the jaundice is prolonged or deep, then referral for investigation is indicated.

The best assessment is that this patient has presented in a manner consistent with hepatitis A. The fact that she is on oral contraceptives and had recently had a tonsillectomy raises other possibilities. This should increase your index of suspicion, and if she does not recover rapidly would indicate referral for further investigation. If serious doubts are pre-sent a domiciliary visit could be used as a means of obtaining further advice. To readmit this patient for further investigation after her recent stay in hospital would be difficult for her and the family, who have made considerable contributions already. Close super-vision and observation at home with bed rest and an assessment of her support network should be urgently undertaken.

She should be advised to discontinue oral contra-ceptive tablets for a period of about a year and other contraceptive measures should be discussed. Her husband and children need to be involved in the management and an estimate made of their attitude to this unexpected event. They may feel that it is a complication of tonsillectomy. It is important to give the patient and her family some sort of prognosis against which they can measure progress. For example, hepatitis A is an inflammation of the liver due to a virus; it is usually mild and the jaundice fades in about 7–10 days. The patient feels ill out of proportion to the degree of jaundice and rest is the most helpful treatment, as it shortens the recovery period. This is a condition which may take several months to resolve completely.

Visit at regular intervals looking for signs of re-solution and repeat the liver function tests in about 3 months. They may take up to about a year to return to normal.

In fact this jaundice subsided rapidly and Mrs Crane-Ley made an uneventful recovery. Her husband was on vacation and was able to look after his wife with the aid of her sister, who lived nearby.

Table 27.2 Serum biochemical tests for the investigation of jaundice

Test	Normal range	Value
Total bilirubin	5–17 μmol/l	Severity of jaundice.
Conjugated ('direct') bilirubin	5 μmol/l	Gilbert's syndrome Haemolysis
Alkaline phosphatase	21–100 IU/l	Mainly raised in obstructive (cholestatic) liver disease, e.g. stones in common bile duct
Gamma glutamyl transpeptidase (gamma GT)	10–48 IU/l	Alcoholism (Liver function tests for alcohol are discussed in Chapter 33.) Cholestasis
Alanine transaminase (ALT)	2–53 IU/l	High if hepatic cell damage e.g. due to hepatitis.
Albumin	30–50 g/l	Normal in acute jaundice; low values in chronic liver disease

TEACHING POINTS

1. When a patient presents with extremely vague symptoms it is necessary to take a formal history and perform a systematic examination (provided that your suspicions are aroused).
2. Infectious hepatitis frequently presents in this way.
3. The causes of jaundice are many. It is wise to refresh your memory.
4. Careful consideration should narrow the diagnostic field.
5. The management decision is based on your working diagnosis.
6. The patient and family need to be carefully briefed.
7. Criteria for referral to hospital should be identified.

28 GIDDINESS

The patient who presents with giddiness, or who admits to it during a consultation, poses a very difficult problem and new entrants to general practice find it hard to manage. The reasons for this are threefold. First, giddiness is a common symptom and is frequently presented to the doctor. Secondly, this complaint gives rise to great difficulties in communication, because what the patient is actually experiencing is often very difficult to ascertain. Thirdly, giddiness may be the first indication of serious disease. How then should it be approached?

As with all vague presenting symptoms, it is helpful to have a framework for dealing with the problem. This consists of an appropriate history and examination and a brief check-list of conditions presenting as giddiness. This will enable a doctor to establish what is being described and to have some knowledge of the likely causes. He should also recognize a time-scale within which the symptom may be assessed.

The *Oxford English Reference Dictionary* defines giddiness as:

1. a sensation of whirling and a tendency to fall or stagger or spin round
2. overexcited, mentally intoxicated
3. excitable frivolous
4. in Old English it meant insane (literally possessed by a god).

It is as well to remember that when a patient uses the word giddiness to describe symptoms he or she may be referring to any of the above definitions, which are, after all, part of linguistic heritage. It is up to the physician to define the terms and communicate with the patient in order to do so.

Fifteen per cent of women and 6% of men have experienced giddiness in the 2-week period prior to a symptomatic enquiry. It is a symptom which occurs twice as often over the age of 65 as it does below. Patients presenting with a disturbance of balance represent 1.3 per 1000 patient contacts and the ratio is two females to one male.

A 60-year-old man, Herbert Dale, presented one evening in the surgery saying that he felt giddy.

How would you approach this problem?

The most important diagnostic step is to divide those who are experiencing some form of sensation in the head from those who are experiencing movement. Vertigo is a subjective sensation of abnormal movement in space, it frequently includes a sensation of rotation and may be associated with nausea and vomiting. It is important to remember that vertigo, and particularly vomiting, are symptoms and not a diagnosis. The first objective should be to establish whether or not the term is being used, therefore, to describe movement. Sensations of floating, light-headedness, or feeling intoxicated are more likely to be associated with conditions outside the ear and labyrinth and are very common. Other questions should include associated noises, the presence or absence of deafness, a brief drug history, family history of deafness, any previous similar episodes, the duration, severity and nature of the attacks, and an enquiry into the patient's perception of the cause.

This patient says that he is having brief attacks of giddiness which consist of the room spinning round for a few moments, and leaving him feeling slightly nauseated. He has had a number of these attacks in the past but they are getting more frequent and he has noticed some recent deafness.

What examination would you now perform?

The general demeanour of the patient will indicate whether his appearance is compatible with his age, and whether there is any evidence of arteriosclerosis (for example, an arcus senilis or xanthomata). Examination of his ears will exclude the presence of wax and a Rinne test may indicate otosclerosis. A negative Rinne test, when the bone conduction is louder than air conduction, in an otherwise normal ear, is strongly suggestive of otosclerosis. A further Weber test may confirm that this is localized and a whispered voice test may also indicate the presence of deafness. Figure 28.1 shows the vestibular apparatus.

A further most important examination is to test for nystagmus. Nystagmus is involuntary rhythmic movement of the eyes. It can be seen as a normal response when someone looks out of a train window at the passing scenery. To test for nystagmus ask the patient to look at your finger held up in front of him (more than 50 cm away from the eye) and then moved slowly to the side. Move the finger left and then right, then up and down slowly—count to 5 before moving your finger as nystagmus can be slow to develop. Avoid moving your hand too far out as jerking movements of the eye can occur at extremes of the field of vision. Remember that nystagmus that is not well sustained may be of doubtful significance. Box 28.1 shows the various causes of nystagmus.

There are three types of nystagmus:

1. pendular

Box 28.1 The causes of nystagmus

1. Physiological (optokinetic) at the extreme of the lateral range of vision
2. Errors of refraction and macular lesions
3. Weakness of the ocular muscles
4. Lesions of the cranial nerves III, IV or VI
5. Brainstem lesions
6. Cerebellar lesions
7. Vestibular lesions
8. High cervical cord lesions
9. Idiopathic or congenital, e.g. benign paroxysmal positional nystagmus

---

2. jerking movements either in a horizontal, vertical or occasionally in a rotary fashion
3. coarse ataxic movements.

By far the most common is a fine nystagmus produced by looking to one side with the fast component indicating the side of the lesion.

For a summary of the causes of giddiness see Box 28.2.

The duration of symptoms in an attack of vertigo is

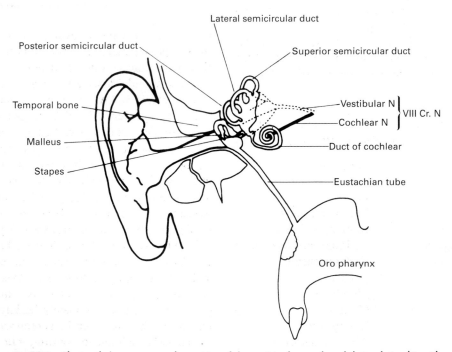

Fig 28.1 The vestibular apparatus, the position of the semicircular canals and their relationship with the middle ear.

Box 28.2 Possible causes of giddiness and their detection

Giddiness may be a term used by patients in any of the following conditions:

1. True vertigo (see Box 28.4)
2. Hypotension or hypertension. (Blood pressure taken standing and sitting)
3. Anaemia. (Pallor, haemoglobin)
4. Intracranial hypertension. (Fundi)
5. Hypoglycaemia. (Enquire into eating habits. Blood sugar—test urine)
6. Epileptic aura. (An appropriate history and past history)
7. Migraine. (A careful history)
8. Psychogenic causes. (Enquire into diet and alcohol and social problems)

Box 28.4 Central nervous system causes of vertigo

1. Vestibular lesions	a. physiological
	b. labyrinthitis
	c. Menière's disease
	d. drugs, e.g. quinine and salicylates
	e. otitis media
	f. motion sickness
	g. benign positional paroxysmal vertigo (BPPV)
2. Vestibular nerve lesions	a. acoustic neuroma
	b. drugs, especially streptomycin
	c. vestibular neuronitis
3. Brainstem, cerebellar or temporal lobe lesions	a. pontine haemorrhage
	b. vertebrobasilar insufficiency
	c. basilar artery migraine
	d. multiple sclerosis
	e. tumours
	f. syringobulbia
	g. temporal lobe epilepsy

important, for many people can experience transient symptoms for a short time. The incidence figures show some 6% of the population may have had this symptom in the recent past. It is therefore important to have some form of management plan for dealing with cases presenting in the surgery.

Box 28.3 shows possible causes of nausea and vomiting which may present as giddiness. Box 28.4 indicates the causes of vertigo.

This list of possibilities serves as a check for those with very persistent symptoms. However, if the examination and the history suggest a vertigo of recent

Box 28.3 Common causes of nausea and vomiting which may or may not be associated with vertigo/giddiness

• ENT	Labyrinthitis
	Menière's disease
	Post surgery
	Motion sickness
• Pregnancy	Morning sickness
• Neurological	Multiple sclerosis
• Biochemical	Hypercalcaemia
• Drugs	Digoxin
	Morphine
• Gastrointestinal	Gastritis
	Biliary disease
	Alcohol ingestion
• Psychological	Eating disorders

onset it is reasonable to treat and wait to see whether the symptom persists. A further follow-up in a week's time will indicate whether treatment has or has not been successful. Most cases of vertigo of benign origin resolve within 3–4 weeks. The flow diagram indicates one such approach. (Fig. 28.2). In general practice the most common causes of vertigo are vestibular neuronitis, labyrinthitis and benign positional paroxysmal vertigo (BPPV). BPPV is worse with head movement and can be confirmed by the Hallpike test, extending and rotating the head through 90°, when vertigo and nystagmus are produced. Treatment of BPPV is by head positioning manoeuvres, e.g. Epley's manoeuvre.

In this patient's case he is describing a series of attacks of giddiness associated with some deafness, and with a family history of deafness; this is suggestive of Menière's disease. As this is a slowly progressive disease, ultimately leading to significant loss of hearing, it would be appropriate to refer him for an ENT opinion to confirm your suspicions. A caloric test and an audiogram would be performed and these would be useful baselines for future

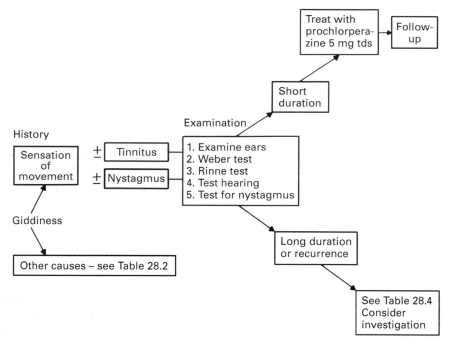

Fig 28.2 Management of giddiness.

Table 28.1 Drugs commonly used for giddiness

Preparation	Dose	Notes
Antihistamines		
Cinnarizine (Stugeron)	30 mg 2 h before travelling, then 8-hourly during journey	Not recommended under 5 years; age 5–12 years, $\frac{1}{2}$ adult dose. Used for vestibular disorders and motion sickness
Promethazine (Avomine)	10–25 mg t.d.s.	Established use in pregnancy and motion sickness
Dimenhydrinate (Dramamine)	50–100 mg 2–3 times a day	7–12 years, $\frac{1}{2}$–1 tablet adult dose; 1–6 years, $\frac{1}{4}$–$\frac{1}{2}$ tablet adult dose; not recommended under 1 year. Used for vertigo, nausea and vomiting, motion sickness
Labyrinthine problems		
Cinnarizine (Stugeron)	15–30 mg t.d.s.	
Prochlorperazine (Stemetil—a phenothiazine)	5–10 mg t.d.s.	Also available as: 12.5 mg injection; 5 or 25 mg suppository and as a buccal preparation (Buccastem 3–6 mg b.d.)

reference. It is also useful to discuss with the patient at this stage the implications of the diagnosis once it has been confirmed. Table 28.1 summarizes drugs commonly used in different types of giddiness.

Some months later you receive a letter from the consultant saying: 'Since I last saw him he has had one episode of vertigo which was worse than any other he has previously experienced. His symptoms are typical of Menière's syndrome and his audiogram and caloric tests support this diagnosis.

TEACHING POINTS

1. A very careful history, and particularly obtaining a description of a sensation of movement, will go far to elucidating the problem.
2. The presence of nystagmus suggests a labyrinthine involvement. Most conditions respond to treatment with either prochlorperazine maleate or cinnarizine.
3. Familiarity with a list of possible causes will avoid omissions in the history.

29 DYSLEXIA

Unfortunately dyslexia is a complicated topic; it is, as yet, not fully understood by any discipline. It can be defined as a specific difficulty in learning, constitutional in origin, which results in significant and permanent difficulty with reading, spelling, written prose, and sometimes arithmetic. It occurs in spite of normal teaching and is independent of intelligence and sociocultural background.

The recognizable collection of signs and symptoms make up the dyslexic syndrome. Also referred to as specific learning difficulty, the terms are often used interchangeably, partly as a result of the move away from 'labelling' by the teaching profession, who prefer specific learning difficulty. This unfortunately leads to parental confusion and reinforces the feeling that the problem has not been understood. Those who suffer from this condition seem to prefer the term dyslexia.

Few of us have any concept of how difficult it is to learn to read and write. Not only do we have to learn to recognize the shape of letters but we have to associate them with sounds. Different combinations of letters are associated with very different sounds (e.g. bough, cough, enough, through, thought, though). This requires more than eyesight and hearing, it requires sophisticated intellectual skills.

When children begin to read at school a group emerge who appear to have greater difficulty than most. There may be many reasons for this but, if there is a specific problem with reading and spelling and it is associated with difficulty in sequencing and orientation, this has been termed *dyslexia* (derived from the Greek word meaning 'difficulty with words'). It is a tragedy for these children that our educational system is based on such skills.

Which children have specific reading difficulties?

It is estimated that nearly 2 million, or 6%, of the adult population of the United Kingdom are illiterate.

Twenty-five per cent of children leaving Infant School have reading difficulty and 10% of those leaving Primary School still have difficulty.

In many the problem is a general retardation of learning; in others there is a 'specific reading delay'. There is a strong association with reading difficulties and later delinquent behaviour. One-third of children with behaviour disorders are thought to have reading problems.

Dyslexia is thought to occur in between 4 and 10% of schoolchildren. Boys are affected more frequently than girls in the ratio of 4 to 1. There is frequently a family history of reading difficulty and a social class gradient.

The problem takes time to emerge and all too often it is not recognized until it is too late to offer constructive help. Early recognition is essential.

Mrs Somerset looked tense and worried as she sat down. 'I've come about Peter,' she said. 'The school are saying that he is difficult to teach and may have dyslexia but I just think he is clumsy. We're all clumsy and I just think that they are not adopting the right approach.'

What is the problem?

The presenting symptoms of dyslexia will include some of the following behaviour patterns

- Difficulty with reading and spelling but it can also present as bad handwriting. There is directional confusion when working with numbers (multiplication tables and directional problems confusing 56 with 65).
- The pronunciation of some words is difficult (crinimal). Frequently b, s and d, s are confused (orientation). The recognition of the sequence in which letters and syllables are placed is impaired ('bread beard'). There is difficulty in distinguishing between certain words (saw was; felt left).

Box 29.1   The features of dyslexia

1. Clumsiness
2. Defective speech
3. Lack of concentration
4. Frustration at own achievements
5. Difficulty with placing letters, words, phrases in reading and writing in the correct sequence
6. Seems 'odd'—different, from other children
7. Poor retention in learning to read new work
8. Tendency to fall easily; accident prone
9. Left-handedness in writing or with tools or signs of ambidexterity
10. Mirror writing
11. Restlessness; hyperactivity
12. Discrepancy between 'brightness' and school progress
13. Normal and or superior spatial and/or motor abilities
14. Persistent disordered spelling even when skills of reading have been acquired
15. Slowness in reading

How does this present?

The reading difficulty.   The first sign is generally slowness in learning to read. The teacher usually notices a discrepancy between the child's ability to read and his ability to answer questions orally. There is an even bigger discrepancy between the oral answers and the written ones.

The handwriting difficulty.   The sequence of letters is often faulty. There may be problems of sequencing events; verbs are often used in the wrong tense or different tenses in the same sentence. The handwriting is often difficult to read, untidy and uneven.

Visual perception.   Dyslexics have difficulty in recalling the shapes of letters and the order in which they come. This extends to groups of letters and words and there is also difficulty in associating a meaning with the written word. The dyslexic's difficulty in learning to read is due to poor perception of symbols and the recognition and recall of letters.

Auditory perception.   Those with poor auditory perception lack the rhythm of language. They cannot clap in time. Like Dr Spooner, they cannot pronounce certain words—'infantry', for example, becomes 'intranfy'.

Sequencing.   When reading it is necessary to get the letters in the correct order. A problem occurs because the dyslexic cannot tackle a word from left to right. They have a similar problem with Arabic, which is sequenced from right to left, or Chinese, which is read top to bottom. Examples of this are typically writing 'was' for 'saw' 'on' for 'no', 'being' for 'begin'.

Orientation.   Letters have to face the correct way. Not only the shape of a letter but the way in which it faces is important—p b; t f; u n; w m; not only does the shape have to be remembered but the orientation determines the sound it makes.

Is there an anatomical basis?

Dyslexia is genetically determined, although this has not yet been clearly identified. Dyslexics invariably have at least one member of the family who has suffered from reading or spelling difficulties (mother, grandfather, etc.). There is frequently a history of cross-laterality (e.g. right eye, left leg dominance). Recent anatomical postmortem studies, magnetic resonance imaging (MRI) and computerized tomography (CT) have identified consistent variations on normal anatomy in the brains of diagnosed dyslexics—these include differences in the relative size of the right planum temporale and also the size of the corpus callosum, through which neurones communicate from one side of the brain to the other. Differences of levels of electrical activity have been demonstrated.

These studies have shown that the brains of those suffering from dyslexia appear to function less well than those who have no difficulty with reading. MRI showed reduced activity in the area linking the angular gyrus, the area responsible for turning images into words, to Wernicke's area, which controls under-standing of words. Broca's area, which is linked to speech, showed signs of overactivity which suggests increased effort to compensate (Proc Nat Acad Sci 1998 study by Yale Medical School).

Developmental dyslexia, often referred to as 'specific learning difficulty', is a disorder of written language. The term developmental is used to distinguish it from disorders of reading and writing (dysgraphia), which are secondary to damage to the brain as after some strokes. Developmental dyslexia commences in childhood and frequently persists into adult life.

It is defined as a severe difficulty with learning to read, spell and write, despite average or above average intelligence and normal schooling. There are two recognized subtypes: developmental dyslexia is the more severe, causing low reading and spelling ages; development dysgraphia, also known as specific spelling retardation, is primarily a disorder of spelling.

How should children with specific reading difficulty be detected?

As this is primarily a learning problem the first suspicions are usually voiced at school, but unfortunately not all teachers recognize it as an entity and this may give rise to difficulties.

Infants. Children often reverse letters at the age of 5 or 6 and cannot always remember the sounds which are represented by certain letters. This usually goes by the age of 7 but with dyslexia this does not happen. Dyslexics are often very reluctant to go to school. The very tearful child, who does not want to go to school or is found truanting, may be showing the first sign that something is amiss.

Young children. By the age of 8 or 9 a dyslexic child is slipping further and further behind. By 8 he may have a reading age of 6.75 years and by 10 may have a reading age of 7.5 years. Should his intelligence be in the 'superior category' his reading age should be well above his chronological age, perhaps by as much as 2 years. His work will have become messy and handwriting cramped and jagged. The spelling may give clues to the problem, as described above. Teachers' remarks often refer to 'poor spelling', 'writing appalling' and he may have gained a reputation as a 'lazy worker'.

Older children. No one copes easily with continual failure and by the age of 11 the dyslexic child with 5 or 6 years of failure behind him tends to opt out. The more intelligent the child, the more frustrating the failure. He often becomes very defensive, has few friends and is afraid to read out loud for fear of ridicule.

How can it be confirmed?

1. The Aston Index. This index comprises a number of specific reading and writing tests. It provides a profile of that child's abilities. Low scores correlate with specific reading retardation and there is a significant difference between dyslexics and other children

with different forms of reading retardation (Thompson & Newton 1975 *Diagnosing dyslexia in the classroom. A preliminary report*, University of London Press).

2. Wechsler Intelligence Scale for Children (WISC). This psychological test is divided into two parts, one to provide evidence of a child's verbal ability and the other to determine his performance ability. There are a number of subsets, one of which is called the Digit Span Sub Test—this is a test of auditory sequencing ability in which dyslexics invariably get a low score.

3. Illinois Test of Psycho-linguistic Abilities (ITPA). This is another psychological test and part of this is the visual sequential memory test. Dyslexics have a very low score on this too.

These tests are administered by educational psychologists and are only described here to illustrate that the features described in dyslexia can be measured using appropriate methods.

The diagnosis of dyslexia is made by an educational psychologist using tests such as the ones described. Referral is usually made through the school but parents may request assessment through their Director of Education or direct from an educational psychologist.

What does the general practitioner do about it?

The role of general practitioners in treating dyslexia is limited but important. Dyslexia is primarily an educational problem but general practitioners have a crucial role to play (Box 29.2). In assessing the child remember the skills required for reading (Box 29.3) and features associated with reading difficulty (Box 29.4).

A general practitioner should be able to identify children who are having language difficulties at an early age and refer them to a speech therapist (Box 29.5). Children whose speech and language difficulties are dealt with in the early years are much less likely to experience reading difficulties when they enter school.

Once dyslexia is considered then an appropriate referral should be made to an educational psychologist.

What can be done about it?

The primary remedy for dyslexia is education. It requires specialist methods that differ substantially from the methods employed in most British classrooms

Box 29.2 The role of the general practitioner

- Recommend appropriate assessment
- Help the family to cope with the emotional problems arising from the child's educational difficulties
- Refer children with speech and language difficulties to speech and language therapists
- Suspect the diagnosis and refer individuals for psychological assessment (usually school educational psychology service (Box 29.3)
- Occasionally schools are unable or unwilling to make such referrals and the general practitioner may be consulted. He or she needs to know how to refer to an appropriate clinical psychologist
- Occasionally parents and teachers have not considered the possible diagnosis
- Failure at school generates much stress in families, sometimes necessitating family therapy (Box 29.4)

Box 29.3 Skills required for reading

1. The ability to understand and use spoken language
2. The ability to recognize a visual symbol
3. They must have normal sound perception and discrimination
4. They must be able to relate written images to oral sounds
5. They require a well-established lateral preference
6. Normal emotional development
7. Normal memory

Box 29.4 Associations of reading difficulties

Reading difficulties are associated with the following:

1. Limited intelligence (low IQ)
2. Low social class
3. Ascending birth order
4. In schools with a high rate of teacher pupil turnover, the use of different methods of teaching
5. Children having to learn in a second language
6. Hearing loss
7. Delays in speech and language development
8. Poor eyesight which may prevent the recognition of certain symbols (but difficulties with visual perception are found less often than those of delayed language development)
9. Left-handedness and cross-laterality may not be associated difficulties but confusion over laterality is
10. Defects in concentration and impulsive behaviour

Note: Reading, writing and spelling problems are often related but not rigidly so; some children can spell words which they cannot read.

and are reminiscent of what would now be regarded as old-fashioned methods: repetition structure and rules learned by rote.

Once a diagnosis has been established the parents must be helped to understand the nature of the condition and several helpful books exist which explain the nature of the condition. The essential thing to understand is that the condition never goes away but that the dyslexic can be taught how to maximize his or her own potential learning ability by employing methods which overcome the inbuilt problems.

New material is presented in small steps and using multisensory pathways, e.g. singing the tables to music. Older children are given instruction in planning their writing of essays and structured study skills. All this requires substantial educational skills and specialist training is required.

An excellent series of booklets is published by the Helen Arkle Dyslexia Centre and can be recommended. Some exercises are designed to overcome difficulties with visual or auditory perception. All approaches depend on an analysis of the child's individual abilities and difficulties. When the diagnosis is established the educational psychologist can issue a certificate, which may be presented to the examination boards, who will make allowances in respect

Box 29.5 Signs to look for

- Late speech development
- Difficulty in naming known objects or people's names
- Persistent word-searching
- Excessive spoonerisms
- Difficulty in learning nursery rhymes, days of the week, months of the year, multiplication tables, etc.
- Often clumsy
- Difficulty throwing, catching, kicking a ball or hopping, skipping and clapping rhythms
- Late learning to fasten buttons or tie shoelaces

Continuing to put shoes on the wrong feet despite the discomfort.

of reading and writing difficulties produced in public examinations.

What do you say to Mrs Somerset?

Parents can be reassured that this is a relatively common problem and the most important step to be taken is to have the condition confirmed by an educational psychologist. It is possible then to institute appropriate teaching techniques to maximize the child's own potential. It is wise at this stage to say that dyslexia is not something which can be cured but that it is a condition which, if recognized, can be helped by appropriate teaching techniques and that there is a large amount of advice and guidance available for parents.

There are special tests which can be used to identify the condition, and referral to an educational psychologist is the best way to get this done. The school may be able to make these arrangements but, if not, then they may be made through the Director of Education. The school is the first point of contact. Drugs have no part to play in the management of this condition but careful assessment and appropriate teaching methods are of considerable help.

What about follow-up?

Following the progress of a dyslexic child is primarily the task of the psychologist and the school but the general practitioner may be involved if the family has difficulties with behaviour or cannot obtain any cooperation at school. Outcome measures are mainly the academic achievements of the children; and on a wider scale the evidence of successful detection would be that the condition would present at an earlier stage and that fewer children would be diagnosed at the age of 10.

Many dyslexics improve dramatically once the diagnosis is made. They need much praise, encouragement and reassurance. Remedial teaching from experts is nearly always required. The eventual prognosis is, of course, determined by individual intelligence and motivation. There is a great tendency for performance to fluctuate on a day-to-day basis and a tendency to regress under the stress of examinations.

At a later stage in the educational process full use should be made of modern technology, typewriters, word processors with spelling checks, and calculators should all be used. It may be that national testing for this condition at the age of 7 will become the norm as more dyslexics are recognized.

Conclusion

Dyslexia is not primarily a medical condition, although it may present to the general practitioner. It is important because early diagnosis and appropriate educational intervention can alter the outcome and reduce the risk of subsequent behavioural difficulties. General practitioners should be aware of the nature of the problem and that there are educational answers to some of the difficulties. Educational psychologists confirm the condition but management depends on cooperation between the school and the parents.

TEACHING POINTS

1. Dyslexia should be suspected when there is an apparent disparity between intelligence and reading ability.
2. The main role of the general practitioner is to exclude medical conditions such as epilepsy.
3. Assessment by an educational psychologist is essential.
4. Parents may need support in coming to terms with the problems.
5. Categorizing the problem as a middle-class excuse for lack of ability is misleading and unhelpful.

FURTHER READING

Dyslexia: a guide for the medical and health care professions. British
  Dyslexia Association
The dyslexia handbook 1998. British Dyslexia Association

Information pack about adult dyslexia. British Dyslexia Association

The British Dyslexia Association is the national charity speaking on behalf of all dyslexics. It provides an information and advisory service, has a help line and publishes brochures and booklets. For more information contact the association at 98 London Road, Reading RG1 5AU (Tel: 0118 966 2677).

30 TERMINAL CARE IN GENERAL PRACTICE

About one-fifth of the population die of cancer and it is estimated that over half of these suffer needless pain. The Health of the Nation strategy identifies cancer as one of its core targets for improved care; not all terminal care given is for patients with cancer. The primary care team will play an increasing role in this task.

Since the first edition of this book there have been significant advances in the provision of care for cancer sufferers and in terminal care. The hospice movement has grown enormously. Specialists in palliative care have emerged as a discipline in their own right. The Marie Curie Welfare Organization and the Macmillan Cancer Relief Fund and its nurses have also expanded. In 1989 the heads of state of governments of the European Community agreed on a European programme against cancer.

Care of the dying is one of the essential tasks for a good doctor. Although only a few patients on a doctor's list will die each year (about 25 deaths a year for a practice population of 2500), the commitment to them means that terminal care is an appreciable part of our work. The support of a dying patient and his or her family can be one of the most worthwhile contributions a doctor can make, and will establish a rapport with the family for many years to come. Conversely, a patient who dies at home with inadequate, irregular visits from a multitude of different doctors and with negligible support of the family is a tragedy for primary care and leaves considerable resentment with the family. As with most other aspects of primary care, the personality of the doctor is as important as the drugs prescribed.

In this chapter we hope to establish some guidelines which will help the doctor in the approach to those with terminal illness. In discussing the subject we must first detail the principles of terminal care outlined below. While terminal care embraces the care of all dying patients, it is exemplified by patients dying of terminal cancer, with whom we are concerned in this chapter.

THE SEVEN PRINCIPLES OF A DOCTOR'S ROLE IN TERMINAL CARE

1. Symptom control and relief (pain, dyspnoea, cough, vomiting, etc.)
2. Communication with the patient—never isolate the patient.
3. Avoidance of inappropriate therapy (infusions, gastrostomy tubes, etc.).
4. Support of the relatives.
5. Teamwork—with nurses, social workers, physiotherapists, etc.
6. Continuity of care—regular visiting by the doctor and nurse
7. Help with bereavement.

1. Symptom control

Ensure that the patient and family are aware that pain will be controlled; there is a great fear of pain and a painful death.

Start analgesia early, regularly and in appropriate dose. Anticipate the next wave of pain by regular dosage.

Do not be afraid of opiates, drug dependency or large doses; give sufficient for the patient's needs.

Know the drugs available well, and be flexible in approach. Most dying patients have difficulty swallowing tablets because of weakness. There comes a time when the oral route gives rise to the danger of aspiration, coughing and dyspnoea. The subcutaneous route is then preferable.

Remember there are other techniques, e.g. nerve blocks. Do not be afraid to consult experts.

Control other symptoms, e.g. constipation, cough, dyspnoea, insomnia. It is important to remember that nausea, giddiness and vomiting can have many causes, e.g. cytotoxic drugs, digoxin, morphine, hypercalcaemia, gastritis, biliary disease.

Instruct patients and family in the use of the drugs; what they are for, what the dosage is, how often they can be given.

Pain is increased by fear, worry, anxiety and depression; treat these as necessary and try to elucidate fears for the patient and for the family. Be unhurried in your approach.

Written instructions are preferable as patients and relatives may forget.

2. Communication

Above all give the patient time to talk of fears and problems.

Be honest and truthful if questioned, but not pessimistically so.

A policy of 'gentle truth' is generally best.

If patients want to know the diagnosis they have a right to; equally they have a right not to know if it is apparent they do not wish to hear the truth.

Adopt a kind, sympathetic approach; do not be afraid to touch the patient.

Take an interest in the patient as a person—past life, hobbies, etc.—not just as a dying patient.

Respect religious convictions.

Never say, 'There is nothing more I can do.'

Don't raise false hopes, but reassure that symptoms will be relieved.

3. Avoidance of inappropriate therapy

Consider the time and question the need for any invasive palliative measures such as intravenous infusions, etc. Respect the patient's wishes.

The drugs needed to prevent distress are:

- analgesics
- anticonvulsants
- hyoscine for 'rattle'
- tranquillizers/antidepressants.

4. Support of the relatives

Help the family in caring for and in communicating with the patient; above all involve them in the patient's care.

Explain the prognosis and symptomatic treatment clearly.

Answer their fears and try to alleviate problems. Do not overlook possibilities of financial help (including attendance allowance).

Stress to them that they are giving help and support that no one else can by allowing the patient to 'die in his or her own bed'.

Give support with nursing problems, etc.

If home care proves impossible do not let them feel a failure.

Try to avoid a 'conspiracy of silence' between family, patient and doctor.

Care does not end with the death of the patient. Visit and support the bereaved.

Try to reduce any feelings of guilt within the family by showing understanding.

5. Teamwork

Involve one or more members of the team, district nurse, health visitor, home help, occupational therapist, social worker, etc; do not forget an appropriate minister of religion.

Get to know the availability of services in your area (e.g. night nursing, laundry services, etc.).

6. Continuity of care

Ensure that the patient and relatives know that someone will always be available night and day to help if needed.

Visit regularly rather than on request only.

Try to ensure as far as possible that it is the same doctor and nurse doing the visiting.

What are the problems of telling the patient the diagnosis and prognosis of the illness? What are the patient's likely reactions to the knowledge that he or she is dying?

There are no hard and fast rules about telling the patient, and every patient is different. An unhurried approach allows a patient time to express fears and usually it becomes not a dramatic 'shall I tell' but slow sharing of the knowledge with the patient. It is never good policy to lie, as the patient will soon lose faith in the doctor, who will be caring for him or her to the end. Nor is it necessary to be blunt; if the patient wishes to know the diagnosis it can be given in a way that is a positive approach, emphasizing that symptoms can be relieved and that some cases do better than others. The hope that he or she will live longer than others with the condition is of benefit and should not be discouraged. Never reinforce hope of recovery when the patient has lost hope and is rapidly deteriorating. The word 'cancer' is particularly horrific to some, and alternatives such as 'growth' somehow seem kinder.

The patient who asks should be told the truth. There are some who do not ask and make it clear that they do not wish to know; this right has to be respected. The relatives should always be told.

There is also the patient who seems unaware of the seriousness of his or her condition (although this may be a denial). As the disease progresses the diagnosis usually becomes obvious.

Much to doctors' surprise most people know their diagnosis long before it is realized that they do; they know by the embarrassment and silence of relatives, friends and doctors, by the sometimes unpleasant treatments, by the look of failure on their doctors' faces and by their own deterioration.

The most difficult situation of all is that in which the patient does not wish the relatives to know or the relatives do not wish the patient to know. This 'conspiracy of silence' makes terminal care exceedingly difficult, and once all realize the situation and the grief and sadness is shared it is generally a relief to all.

A general approach is, therefore, to be unhurried and give the patient time, to be truthful if the patient wishes and to involve the relatives as early as possible. The best drug a patient can be given is the time of doctors, relatives and friends.

To appreciate the patient's reactions to dying and aid the doctor in his or her approach, it is useful to know some of the common fears which the patient may need to discuss. The feelings of resentment and loneliness, and that he or she does not matter any more, are natural; some patients will become aggressive. In contrast there are some who will greet the news with what amounts to pleasure, especially those with deep religious convictions or chronic illness. Common fears include:

1. Fear of the process of dying—will it be painful? Will my symptoms be relieved? The doctor should be able to reassure that symptoms will be controlled.
2. Fear of the unknown and what happens after

death. The whole of the fear of the unknown is intimately bound up with that of the patient's religious convictions, which should be respected. An appropriate Minister of Religion can be invaluable. Some fears, hallucinations or deliriums will be part of a depressive state.
3. Fear of separation from family, house and job, and the consequences for the family. Everything should be done to give assistance with the dying patient's provision for the family; if they will be exposed to severe hardship then social workers may be useful to reassure and help.
4. Fear of depending on others. Reassure that all that can be done to help will be done.

Finally a word on euthanasia. In these days patients need not suffer a painful protracted death, and a cry for euthanasia may be a cry for better relief of symptoms which should be appropriately treated.

During the course of a terminal illness, several stages of adjustment are gone through by the patient, the relatives and indeed the doctor. These are summarized in Table 30.1.

What are the important points to bear in mind when adopting a strategy to relieve pain from terminal cancer?

Pain relief is often poor and at least a quarter of those dying of malignant disease in home and in hospital do so in appreciable pain. Pain is not always present in death from malignancy and indeed 50% have no pain at all. It is virtually always possible to relieve physical pain, but the experience is intimately tied up with mental, social and spiritual factors; attendance to these problems will lower the need for analgesia. If fear and anxiety are major components then a sedative may be necessary.

When confronted with a patient with a malignancy who is in pain, do not always assume the pain is from malignant deposits; always look at the area of the pain, which may reveal bed sores, thrombosed piles, etc., for which other therapy may be appropriate. Antibiotics may be needed for a urinary tract infection or an infected discharge. Bowel colic may require antispasmodics, and constipation should be treated. Dexamethasone may improve symptoms of raised intracranial pressure, at least initially. The use of adjuvant therapy will thus help management considerably.

Table 30.1 Stages of adjustment in terminal illness

	Patient	Relatives	Doctor
1. Denial	'It can't be true' 'It's a mistake' 'It's not really happening'	As patient	'It can't happen to my patient'
2. Anger	'How could this happen to me?' 'What have I done to deserve it?' 'Someone's to blame, probably the doctor'	'How could medicine fail to help?' 'Who is responsible?'	'Why didn't he give up smoking?' 'He should have come to see us much earlier'
3. Bargaining	'Perhaps if I had taken those tablets' 'Perhaps if I had prayed regularly' 'Perhaps if I had given up smoking'	As patient	'How could I have missed the diagnosis? —perhaps if I had ordered a chest X-ray'. ...'Maybe if I had had a domiciliary by a consultant...'
4. Depression	'It really is true' 'What am I going to do?' 'What is going to happen to my family?'	As patient	'I've got to cope with this'
5. Acceptance	'Life goes on' 'I must prepare for my family'	As patient	'I will look after and care for him in his terminal illness to the best of my ability'

There is little place for 'on-demand' analgesia; it must be given regularly. The half-life of most of the more powerful analgesics, e.g. diamorphine, is short and after 4 hours the concentration will have fallen to an inadequate level—hence 4-hourly is the frequency of choice. Using a 4-hourly system we are giving analgesia when some may still be present, thus preventing a breakthrough of pain. With the fear of pain gradually abolished the dosage needed may become less. If pain does recur the dose can be increased, titrating the dose against the pain. In addition to the regular medication the patient can be prescribed extra analgesia for times when the pain does occur in the interval between doses, and this is one strategy that may help to reduce the total amount of opiate and hence sedation. If these extras are being used too often the dose of opiate will have to be readjusted. The policy must be entirely flexible; problems of tolerance and addiction are rarely important in practice, and it needs emphasizing that one of the most common mistakes in pain relief is to use opiates too late and in inadequate dosage.

In this age of specialization pain clinics are an increasing feature of medical life and have much help to offer in difficult cases. Local injections and nerve blocks are useful in selected patients and the technique of intrathecal phenol block can have dramatic effects in pain relief (e.g. a coeliac plexus block for the pain of carcinoma of the stomach or pancreas). When pain control is poor do not hesitate to seek advice on other methods. Local heat, cooling sprays, fixation of joints, drainage of ascites; all these may be appreciated by individual patients. Palliative surgery may very occasionally be necessary, for example in relieving an acute bowel obstruction.

Outline a hierarchy of analgesics to control pain from malignant disease in a patient dying at home.

Table 30.2 lists a hierarchy of analgesia.

Note that for severe pain, morphine is best. The Oramorph solutions are useful preparations here, coming in a standard strength of 2 mg/ml and Oramorph concentrated at 20 mg/ml. A phenothiazine syrup, however, is useful as an antiemetic and tranquillizer. At first, adjust the morphine dose, then add the phenothiazine. Of the phenothiazines, prochlorperazine syrup (Stemetil) is less sedative, but chlorpromazine syrup (Largactil) can be used if additional sedation is required. Other agents used to manage vomiting include haloperidol and metoclopramide. There are various ways of delivering morphine and a great advance has been the continuous infusion system using syringe pumps. These often enable a patient to remain at home, pain-free, for considerably longer than may otherwise have been the case.

Other useful analgesic strategies in controlling chronic severe cancer pain are:

1. Use of fentanyl patches—these come in 25–100 µg

Table 30.2 Analgesics in terminal disease

	Analgesic	Comments
Mild-pain	Aspirin Paracetamol	Use regularly. Beware of gastrointestinal effects of aspirin
Mild to moderate pain	Dihydrocodeine Coproxamol Various codeine preparations	Note that pethidine is probably too short-acting to be useful and may give unpleasant nausea. Pentazocine (Fortral) is also of limited usefulness. If metastases in bone, add prostaglandin synthetase inhibitors, e.g. Naproxen
Moderate to severe pain	Dextromoramide (Palfium) Dipipanone plus cyclizine (Diconal) Phenazocine (Narphen) Buprenorphine (Temgesic) Tramadol (Zamadol, Zydol)	The action of dextromoramide is only adequate for about 2 hours but is useful for exacerbation of pain. Buprenorphine can cause dependence, and vomiting may be a problem. Tramadol has a particular advantage in having an opioid-like action but without significant respiratory depression or constipation. In severe pain of any degree resort to morphine, but these are useful aids
Severe pain	Morphine preparations	Oramorph is a useful solution; MST is a sustained-release oral tablet. Diamorphine is for injection. A continuous infusion via a syringe pump is a very effective way of delivering morphine

and each patch lasts 72 hours. Said to provide continuous pain relief similar to morphine.
2. Use of oxycodone suppositories—particularly useful if the patient cannot tolerate the oral route.

Consider the advantages and disadvantages of trying to manage a dying patient at home. What are the alternatives to home care?

The very best and the worst of terminal care can occur at home. About one-third of patients die at home, two-thirds in hospital and 5% in non-NHS hospitals or hospices. Some of these hospital deaths, however, will be only days after admission, the general practitioner having cared for the patient prior to admission.

It is not useful to make dogmatic assertions that all patients should die at home, or indeed in hospices; much depends on the individual and the circumstances at the time. In fact a dying patient may spend part of the terminal illness at home and part in hospital. Let us consider the alternatives.

1. Home. Most patients would probably like to die in familiar surroundings and the relatives may feel a failure if they cannot cope with this. There are four factors that usually determine whether home care is feasible:

a. *The patient*
   Does he or she wish to? (Some feel they will be too great a burden to their families.)
   Does he or she need constant nursing care?
   Are there any important medical needs that can only be received in hospital?

b. *The relatives*
   How many are there?
   Do they live with the patient or a long way away?
   Do they feel they can cope?
   What is their financial position; do they work full-time?
   Has an attendance allowance been applied for?
   Can they look after the patient at night?

c. *The services available*
   Are home helps available?
   Is there an incontinent laundry service if needed?
   Are night nurses available?
   Are bedpans, commodes, etc. available?

d. *The practice team*
   Availability of members of the team, e.g. district nurses.
   Presence or absence of a night nursing service, and nursing cover at weekends.

2. Hospital. Care may often fall below desirable levels here for a variety of reasons. Sometimes death is regarded as a failure and patients are moved to side wards and passed rapidly by on ward rounds. The staff may be busy and the patients apologetic for taking up so much valuable time. Analgesia should be no problem, but an alarmingly high proportion of patients still die in pain even in hospital.

3. Hospice/terminal care unit. Hospices specializing in terminal care are few in number, but a visit to one should be part of every doctor's education. The staff are specialists in symptom control and a positive commitment to the patients with an individual approach ensures some of the very best of terminal care. There are few spaces in these units but day care in them is increasingly common. Their value as a training centre for doctors and nurses is great.

7. Help with bereavement

The care of the grieving relatives is just as much a responsibility for the doctor as the care of the dying patient. During the care of the dying patient the doctor has an opportunity to build up a good rapport with the relatives. A visit by the doctor after the death is invaluable, with the promise that support will be available if needed; this equally applies if the patient has died in hospital. Grief reactions are very varied in their manifestations and in particular delayed grief reactions can be very distressing. A bereaved person who acts as if nothing has happened may be heading for a very severe emotional grief reaction. Sedatives may be useful, but the most valuable service to the bereaved is the support of relatives, neighbours and friends. Rehabilitation can be made easier by the encouragement of the bereaved person's interests, and a holiday may be therapeutic. A common problem is for the bereaved to ask the doctor's advice; for instance, should they sell their home and move. Here the utmost caution should be exercised.

Home care of the terminally ill is very valuable preparation for bereavement, and at least one study shows that mortality among the bereaved is less if the death occurred at home.

TEACHING POINTS

1. Terminal care is one of the most important areas of general practice.
2. Revise the seven principles of terminal care.
3. Analgesia must be regular and appropriate. Morphine is best for severe pain.
4. A kind, caring approach by the doctor is as beneficial as the medication he or she prescribes.
5. The care of the grieving relatives is very important; terminal care does not end with the death of the patient.

31 PROBLEMS WITH BABIES

Child care forms a quarter of all general practice and a very important quarter it is. It is an essential part of good general practice and patients seem to get to know which doctor in a practice is good with children. Paediatrics is also a danger area for the inexperienced—illnesses such as epiglottitis and meningitis can develop rapidly and fatally and the penalties for missing such an illness are grave; even relatively common illnesses such as gastroenteritis may be serious. A great deal of knowledge is required by the general practitioner, not least in the areas of immunization, developmental assessment and infant feeding. All doctors dealing with children should have an ample supply of growth charts to plot a child's weight, length and head circumference, as detection of failure to thrive is an essential part of the general practitioner's role. Good health visitors will be worth their weight in gold to a practice and will deal with many of these problems, but a sound knowledge, and confidence in dealing with babies and the anxieties of a worried mother, will make paediatric practice an enjoyable part of a doctor's life.

NAPPY RASH

General practitioners see and advise many mothers about one of the most common of infantile problems, which is nappy rash. Most are easy to manage, but some can be a difficult problem to treat, and even hospital referral may be needed if the features are unusual.

Mrs Mills brought her 5-week-old Matthew to the surgery frequently in the first weeks of his life, despite advice from the health visitor and her own mother. He did however have quite a severe nappy rash extending over the buttocks, upper thighs and genitalia.

What does the normal nappy rash look like, and what other causes are there of a rash in this area?

The common *simple napkin dermatitis* (*ammoniacal dermatitis*) is usually not hard to diagnose, presenting in its mildest form as an erythema over the areas of closest contact with the wet napkins, i.e. the buttocks, inner upper thighs, genitalia and lower abdomen. The skin creases, which do not come into contact with the wet nappy, are characteristically spared. Severe cases may present with vesicles, papules, erosions and ulceration, which soon becomes infected. Infection with *Candida* is important to recognize and presents as moist red patches with a raised scaling edge and satellite lesions; it involves the skin creases and may spread from the perianal region. A *seborrhoeic 'eczematous' form* of napkin rash is recognized as a diffuse rash in the nappy areas often associated with other indications of a seborrhoeic dermatitis, e.g. grey scaling of the scalp and involvement of other flexures including axillae and neck: *Napkin psoriasis*, with sharply marginated red scaly plaques, affects other areas of the body; few of these children develop true psoriasis in later life. A *perianal rash* may be due to persistent loose stools. The rarer lesions each have their own characteristic associations, e.g. diarrhoea and weight loss with *acrodermatitis enteropathica*. *Atopic dermatitis* (*infantile eczema*) as such is seldom seen before 3 months and usually starts on the forehead and cheeks. Table 31.1 indicates which of these conditions are relatively common.

What are the predisposing factors to simple napkin dermatitis?

The classical view of the common nappy rash was that it was due to ammonia liberated from urea in the urine by urease activity of certain bacteria. Research has not wholly supported this view and the chief factors seem to be infrequent changes of wet nappies allowing

Table 31.1 Eruptions in the napkin area

Relatively common	Others
Napkin dermatitis (ammoniacal dermatitis)	Napkin psoriasis
	Congenital syphilis
	Acrodermatitis enteropathica
Seborrhoeic dermatitis	Letterer–Siwe disease
Candidiasis	Herpes simplex
	Impetigo
	Intertrigo
	Miliaria

prolonged contact with skin, the use of tight fitting rubber or plastic pants, infection, and an increased sensitivity of the skin in some babies. Sensitivity to some detergents may also be a problem.

How would you treat Matthew's nappy rash?

A major improvement in the rash will be effected by the simple measure of exposing the area and leaving the baby lying on a nappy rather than wrapped in it. Nappies should be changed frequently. Having removed a wet nappy the skin should be washed with water, dried and light talcum powder applied. Barrier creams are effective in prevention, e.g. zinc and castor oil cream, Drapolene, dimethicone-containing preparations, and old-fashioned egg white. Waterproof airtight plastic and rubber pants should be abolished. There are now special polypropylene one-way nappies which limit the amount of urine next to the skin and specially absorbent ones.

If infection with *Candida albicans* is suspected or the rash does not respond to the above therapy in about 10 days, try a nystatin preparation, e.g. Nystaform HC. If *Candida* is present, also look in the mouth for oral candidiasis. Note that there is no place for fluorinated topical steroids in the treatment of nappy rash. Seborrhoeic dermatitis responds to 1% hydrocortisone.

CONSTIPATION

Perhaps more than any other function the regulation of the bowels is regarded as of prime importance by patients, and mothers are no exception.

Gillian Green had a bonny 5-week-old infant whom she was breast-feeding. She was worried that it was *nearly 2 days since he had passed a stool and wondered if I could give him something to 'loosen him up'.*

What do you think of this problem?

The most important point here is the understanding of what is normal. Stool frequency is very variable among babies; breast-fed babies especially may vary in the frequency with which they pass stools, from one after each feed to one every 7–10 days. Stools of bottle-fed babies are harder and often passed every day; with underfeeding, small firm green 'hunger' stools may be produced, sometimes accompanied by traces of blood and mucus. Occasionally the passage of dry hard stools by a bottle-fed baby will be a problem; suitable advice would be to increase the water intake either between feeds or by adding a little to each feed. Milk of magnesia (magnesium hydroxide mixture BP) is often effective when this advice fails. The maximum dose for a baby is 10 ml daily. There is no place for laxatives.

If constipation does persist or is associated with intermittent diarrhoea, with vomiting, abdominal distension or with failure to thrive, one must remember other causes of constipation and particularly Hirschsprung's disease, which may be fatal. It has, however, been calculated that an average general practitioner may have to wait 600 years before seeing a new case! The other causes listed in Box 31.1 are uncommon and

Box 31.1 Causes to be considered if constipation persists in babies

1. Mother incorrectly describing symptoms as constipation
2. After a febrile illness
3. Underfeeding and too little fluid intake
4. Anal anomaly, e.g. stenosis, stricture, malposition
5. Spinal anomaly such as spina bifida
6. Hypothyroidism
7. Hypercalcaemia
8. Coeliac disease can present as constipation after the introduction of gluten-containing food into the diet
9. Hirschsprung's disease

the anatomical abnormalities should have been picked up at birth. The management of 'constipated' babies thus revolves around a good feeding history and health education of the mother.

A CRYING BABY

All babies cry but some cry more than others. Similarly some mothers tolerate crying in their baby more than others. There are many reasons why a crying baby may be brought to the surgery and any list would be enormous. Some mothers feel their baby is abnormal in that he cries so much. Some mothers come because they expect the baby not to cry and in particular because it disturbs family sleep; it can, however, be a real problem, as any tired and exhausted parent can testify. A mother may come into the surgery in sheer desperation with her baby, and then the possibility of non-accidental injury must be borne in mind.

Jean Forrest was married to a builder's labourer and they had a 3-month-old son called David. 'I just can't stand him crying any more,' she said. It transpired that the baby did cry a lot, especially at night when her husband was trying to sleep, and he was not the most tolerant of fellows. The baby was not placated by a feed, and Jean could only quieten him by cuddling him up to her, when he would fall off to sleep again. The baby was in a cot in the room next to the parents.

What are the causes of a crying baby?

There are of course many causes and Table 31.2 lists most of them. In fact, it is unusual to find a cause, and the problem usually resolves spontaneously with time. Just as with other illnesses, the history is all important. The first point to establish is the length of the history, i.e. is this a normal baby who has suddenly had bouts of screaming and crying or is the history a longer one? The usual investigatory questions about a symptom apply to 'crying', i.e. when does it occur, aggravating and relieving factors, associated symptoms, etc. Note that in babies the feeding history is of special importance—an unwell baby does not feed well. Social background and knowledge of the family and housing conditions will be valuable and the health visitor may contribute much to the discussion and

Table 31.2 Crying in babies: some causes and advice

Cause	Advice
1. Hunger	Many babies cry when a feed is due. Some babies need to be fed more frequently than 3-hourly. Feed times may need to be adjusted and some babies need their night feed longer than others. Some mothers recognize a 'hunger cry'
2. Thirst	Giving extra water may solve this; it is worth a try offering some water twice a day. A drink of water may be offered instead of an extra bottle
3. Emotional causes	Babies and infants like to be with their mothers and like the warmth of contact; picking them up may stop the crying. A harness to the mother is useful. Firm wrapping in a cot gives contact and sucking a dummy helps. A few soft toys may distract attention in older infants. Sleeping in the same room as mother may have a quieting effect
4. Abuse or neglect	
5. Organic illness	Persistent screaming and crying may be the first sign of an infection, e.g. otitis media or urinary tract infection. There will usually be other symptoms—check if the baby is feeding well, gaining weight, etc. Intussusception may present as repeated screaming attacks increasing in frequency during the day. Look also for a hernia
6. Napkin irritation	Some napkins are left on too long and may be wet and soiled
7. Feeding problems	
8. 'Three months' or 'evening colic'	Classically in the evening after the 6 p.m. feed the baby draws the legs up and screams. The attacks usually disappear after 3 months. Activated dimethacone (Infacol) may help (0.5–1 ml before feeds)
9. ?Nightmares	
10. ?Teething	Probably *not* a cause. Think again!
11. ?Lack of stimulation	

further management. Signs of neglect and failure to thrive may indicate a poor mother–infant relationship as much as organic illness. Organic illness should be excluded and is unlikely with a long history when the baby is feeding well, his growth following the percentiles and developing normally. Crying may be the first sign of an infection if there is an acute change, and the infant should be examined thoroughly and other symptoms (diarrhoea, vomiting, etc.) rigorously enquired about. Remember in particular intussusception as a cause of acute screaming attacks. Reassurance that all is well with the baby may be all that is required, and sometimes a baby-minder to give the parents a night off occasionally can also work wonders. Changing milks is very unlikely to make any difference and there is nothing worse than seeing a mother advised various different milks by different people.

In the case of Mrs Forrest I was well acquainted with the family situation. The husband was unemployed. He occasionally used to beat his wife, and they were living in poor conditions on a large housing estate with little support. When I examined the baby I could find nothing abnormal; he was feeding well and his length, weight and head circumference were all near the 50th centile. The mother was quite distressed. Having examined the child I leaned forward to talk to her. I was particularly concerned, knowing the family and particularly the father, that this was a baby who was in danger of being battered.

There is much to be gained by gently exploring this area sympathetically. Use questions such as 'You must feel pretty desperate' or 'You must find it very difficult to cope.' The answer to these questions will allow parents the opportunity to vent their anger and guilt without feeling persecuted. The vast majority will respond to reassurance and sympathy.

In this case I was very concerned and so was the health visitor. The family had reached a 'crisis point' over the baby's crying and I felt that, in everybody's interest, a brief admission to hospital would be justified to defuse the situation. I talked to the paediatrician and this was arranged. On discharge from hospital it goes without saying that the baby was closely followed by myself and the health visitor.

A good liaison between hospital paediatrician and general practitioner is invaluable in these tense situations, but this is, of course, a very exceptional case.

IS MY BABY GETTING ENOUGH MILK?

This heartfelt plea is all too common in the pursuit of the largest and 'bonniest' baby; all too often the answer is that the baby is receiving too much!

Barbara Williams, a London graduate married to an accountant, was a mother who believed her 2-month-old baby was not getting enough milk. The baby was being bottle-fed and she brought him with his bottle to the surgery. The practice has, in fact, an excellent team of health visitors who do answer many of the mothers' queries; but this particular mother had an obsessional personality and was prone to reading textbooks on infant care. I approached the consultation with trepidation as I was sure she would already have read widely about the problem.

Every general practitioner should be able to advise on infant feeding problems and answer all the common questions mothers ask. In most cases reassurance is all that is necessary. The involvement of the health visitor at this stage is important. Once again it is stressed that the plotting of weight, length and head circumference is not only the province of hospital paediatricians. Child health record cards contain centile charts and it can be most reassuring to show these to the mother, as I did on this occasion: her baby was growing perfectly well along the 50th centile. A welcome move recently has been the introduction of a standardized Personal Child Health Record (the now familiar red booklet issued at birth, produced by the British Paediatric Association in 1992 and now widely adopted throughout the country).

With feeding problems the other major helpful approach is to watch the mother feeding the baby. If he is being bottle-fed, watch the mother make up his feed. This mother was in fact quite expert in these matters, but it can often be very revealing; modern feeds are precisely formulated, so that following the manufacturer's instructions is essential.

There will be a few babies who will not be receiving enough milk, either due to failure of lactation by the mother or because the baby cannot feed well for some reason. Failure of lactation is probably the most common cause of failure to thrive in breast-fed babies. Signs and symptoms of underfeeding include poor weight gain, restlessness with excessive crying, small green 'hunger' stools, and gulping at feeds with mouthing at the end of a feed. The babies should be fully examined and centiles plotted. There is no need to panic because, as long as the baby is well and adequately hydrated, a few days' underfeeding will do no harm. Test feeding is very worrying for the mother.

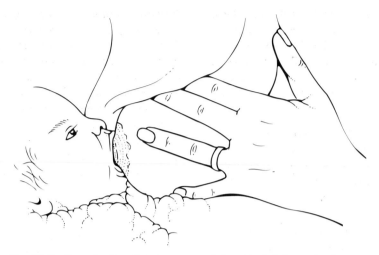

Fig. 31.1 Breast-feeding. Note the correct technique. The baby's nose has been kept clear by gentle pressure on the breast.

At the end of the day there will be some babies who will need complementary feeds, but the doctor should always encourage breast-feeding if at all possible, as long as the mother is able and willing to do so.

This is a suitable point to revise your knowledge

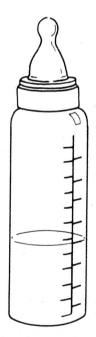

Fig. 31.2 Bottle-feeding. The newer plastic bottles are very suitable. With any feeding problems check the flow of milk from the teat (see text).

about breast-feeding and bottle-feeding (Figures 31.1 and 31.2). Six common questions mothers ask are listed in Table 31.3.

Breast-feeding: advantages

Breast-feeding gives a baby the best start in life (Box 31.2) and also has benefits for the mother (Box 31.3). It not only provides everything needed for a healthy, nutritious and balanced diet but it also helps protect the baby against certain diseases of childhood and in later life. Over half the mothers who start breast-feeding have stopped by 6 weeks—the reasons may vary but many of them can be overcome by sensitive encouragement and support. Reassure mothers that they are providing their babies with the best start in life.

Many women abandon breast-feeding too early because of problems with incorrect positioning of the baby at the breast (Fig. 31.1). The two most common reasons given are that their breasts are painful and they are afraid that they are not giving their babies enough. Both arise from incorrect positioning on the breast, causing nipple trauma and ineffective feeding (Campbell 1997).

The problems of poor positioning are:

- for the mother: sore nipples, breast engorgement and breast abscesses
- for the baby: inadequate feeds, restlessness

Table 31.3 Feeding problems: questions mothers ask

Problem	Advice and notes
1. Are my breasts too small to breast-feed?	Breast size should not matter
2. Is my baby taking enough milk from me? (See also text.)	Check weight gain and signs of underfeeding. Try putting baby to breast more often. Check feeding technique. May need a test feed. Is there any other cause of failure to thrive? Is the baby well?
3. When should I wean my baby?	Solid foods should be introduced from about 4 months; the breast or bottle feeds being tailed off slowly
4. My baby seems to bring up a lot of wind. Is this normal?	Air-swallowing can be due to many causes: a. a baby crying excessively before feeds; b. in 'greedy' feeders who gulp air with their first mouthful of milk (can be helped by spoon-feeding before start of main feed); c. air sucked from the bottle if it is not properly inverted; d. too small a hole in the teat (draws air round teat); e. too large a teat (baby gulps)
5. My baby vomits with most feeds. Why?	What does the mother mean by vomiting? Many babies regurgitate partially digested milk after feeds and enjoy it! The baby gains weight and is well. Sudden true vomiting heralds illness, e.g. an infection or a bowel obstruction. Pyloric stenosis with projectile vomiting is not so uncommon. Chronic vomiting with failure to thrive needs full investigation
6. My baby is feeding very slowly and will not take his feeds. Why?	A baby who suddenly becomes reluctant to feed is usually an unwell baby. One of the more common reasons is an upper respiratory tract infection with blocked nostrils; then ephedrine nose drops 0.5% before feeds may help. Candidiasis in the mouth may be a reason: it should respond to nystatin suspension. The length of time a baby takes to feed is a good indication of the health of that baby

Box 31.2 Benefits of breast feeding—the infant

1. Reduces the risk of babies developing:
   a. gastrointestinal illness
   b. infections of: i. the middle ear
                    ii. respiratory system
                    iii. urinary tract
2. Is associated with reduced risk later in childhood of:
   a. insulin-dependent diabetes
   b. allergies such as eczema
3. For preterm babies, breast milk:
   a. promotes optimum neurological development
   b. reduces the risk of necrotizing enterocolitis
4. The infant is less likely to develop cow's milk protein sensitivity.
5. May provide some protection against cot death.

Box 31.3 Benefits of breast-feeding—the mother

- Reduced risk of premenopausal breast cancer
- Reduced risk of some forms of ovarian cancer
- Social gains: ready available feeding for the baby
- Unique mother–baby contact
- Helps the mother to lose weight naturally

the mouth with the chin close against the breast if the breasts are large; the baby's mouth will not be fully visible but the cheeks will be fully rounded not indrawn. There should be no maternal discomfort.

Disadvantages

1. May not be enough for small-for-dates infant.
2. Cracked nipples caused by faulty latching.
3. There are some contraindications, such as the ingestion of certain drugs by the mother, e.g. lithium.
4. A few mothers cannot produce enough milk.
5. Occasionally infection may occur via this route e.g. transmission of HIV infection has been reported via breast milk.

leading to constant feeding, poor weight gain. When the baby is correctly attached, the angle at the corner of the mouth will be >90°; both lips will be curled back; the nipple will be well within

So what happens in reality? Of 64% who breast-feed at birth, 12% will stop before leaving hospital, 20% will have stopped by 2 weeks, and by 6 weeks only 40% are breast-feeding. All those working in the NHS should promote breast-feeding.

Breast-fed babies do tend to require more frequent feeding than bottle-fed babies. The recommendation is to allow the baby to suck at the breast until he comes off the breast of his own accord with no restriction on the length of time feeding. This allows the baby to have the watery lactose-rich foremilk as well as the fatty calorie-laden hindmilk. If the baby still seems to want to feed he should be offered the second breast. Most babies tend to settle at about a 3-hour schedule. By the end of the first week babies will settle down to one or two night feeds, and after about 6 weeks most babies, but not all, will have omitted the night feed. Most authorities would recommend vitamin and iron supplements (no iron supplements until about 2 months).

Bottle-feeding

1. Use the newer low-solute preparations (e.g. Cow and Gate Premium. SMA Gold Cap). Most milks are fortified with iron and vitamins, so the babies need less vitamin supplementation (but still advisable).

2. The powder must be measured accurately according to instructions with no packed or extra scoops. It is usually 30 ml (1 fl. oz) water: 1 scoop.

3. Check the hole in the teat to give a steady flow of drops from the bottle but not a stream.

4. Sterilize the bottles correctly by boiling or with chemicals.

5. Store in a refrigerator if feeds are made up before use, warming only a few minutes before a feed.

6. Feeds are given on demand or 3–4 hourly. In warm weather give extra water in addition.

7. After the first week of life an average infant will require about 150 ml/kg/day (2½ oz/lb/day).

CHILD HEALTH SURVEILLANCE

The introduction of formal Child Health Surveillance in the 1990 contract has radically altered the care offered to children. This has resulted in general practitioners having special training in monitoring normal children and most practices now offer formal Child Health Surveillance Clinics. The health visitors play a central role in this and general practitioners demonstrate that they have acquired special skills by being placed on the local Child Health Surveillance list. Experience appropriate for this is offered to all registrars. There is now a parent-held child development record in which all routine checks are recorded. Referral pathways for any child found to fail the required development standard are readily available.

TEACHING POINTS

1. Revise the causes of a nappy rash, distinguishing between a simple napkin dermatitis and a candidiasis of the napkin area.
2. Frequent changing of nappies and exposure to air are the most important factors in treating a simple napkin dermatitis.
3. In managing problems with babies, assess the mother's expectation and knowledge.
4. Take a full history as you would for an adult but remember especially with babies the feeding history and their development. The practice should possess centile charts for height, weight and head circumference.
5. The health visitor can be a powerful ally.
6. Encourage mothers to breast-feed their babies whenever possible.
7. Understand the basic problems of infant feeding so that you can help mothers with any problems that may arise.
8. Increasing numbers of women are choosing to breast-feed but many give up during the early weeks; the chief reasons are difficulty in producing milk and discomfort. Both these problems can be rectified by correct positioning of the baby at the breast

FURTHER READING

Campbell C M A V 1997 Early breast feeding failure. *Update* 19 November
National Breastfeeding Working group 1995 *Breastfeeding: good practice guidance to the NHS*. Department of Health, London

32 ANTICIPATORY CARE OF SOME CHRONIC CONDITIONS

In the management of chronic disease each doctor hopes that they are caring for each patient in the best way, balancing the need to identify and prevent possible complications against the intrusion that this makes into the patient's freedom to live life as he or she wishes. In other words doctors try to strike an optimum balance. To do this they need to have a very clear idea what it is they are trying to achieve and what priorities they accept.

Guidelines and their production, for some time a growth industry, is a concept whose time has come. Evidence-based guidelines will dominate the delivery of primary care for the foreseeable future. The new contract introduced by the Labour Government in 1998 placed special emphasis on clinical standards: 'Clinical standards will be monitored and maintained.' It goes on to say that evidence-based frameworks in each disease area will tell patients what they can expect from the NHS. This clearly heralds the introduction of protocols and guidelines that will influence the management of many conditions. The first question to ask, therefore, is whether guidelines exist. In the absence of guidelines questions that should be asked are suggested in Box 32.1; clearly this task will be much easier if a good set of realistic guidelines exists.

What are guidelines and what do they do?

- Practice guidelines are systematically developed statements to assist the practitioner to make appropriate health care decisions.
  - The introduction of guidelines can change clinical practice.
    - They should be based on valid scientific evidence.
    - They should be seen to be suitably authoritative.

Advantages of guidelines
- They provide useful summaries based on good evidence to busy clinicians.

Box 32.1 Questions to ask about a chronic disease

1. What diagnosis has been established?
2. Do criteria for this diagnosis exist?
3. To what extent does this patient fit the known criteria?
4. What prognostic information is available?
5. What therapeutic goals have been identified?
6. Who is responsible for changes in management?
7. What is the natural history of this condition?
8. How can it be modified?
9. What treatments are available and have they any side-effects?
10. What guidelines exist? Are they evidence-based? Do they lead to protocols?

- They are a useful way for generalists and specialists to agree on appropriate management.
- They are a means for an under-recognized speciality to contribute to improving care.
- They can be useful for justifying increased expenditure on effective treatments.
- They can help to reduce wastage and inappropriate methods of treatment.

What is the case against guidelines?
- Scepticism about their ability to achieve any significant clinical change.
- The possibility that they will encourage litigation.
- The reduction of clinical freedom.
- They will produce 'cookbook medicine' or 'medicine by numbers'.
- They will stifle innovation.
- 'I don't trust anyone to do it impartially' says one respected course organizer.

Guidelines have suffered much harm in the past

by appearing as ex-cathedra statements, often by specialists with little knowledge of general practice. Fortunately there is now a readily available source which will indicate whether guidelines have been produced, by whom and whether they have been submitted to the newly proposed National Institute of Clinical Excellence (NICE). National and European Guidelines are included. ('Guidelines—summarising clinical guidelines for primary care' independently produced handbook by Medendium, Publishing Manager, G. Foord-Kelcey.) At present most professional body guidelines remain the property of those who develop them and are not submitted to the Clinical Outcomes Group. Those systematic reviews and guidelines which are prioritized and approved by the Clinical Outcomes Group have been commended by the NHS Executive. For the first time general practitioners will be expected to follow centrally set guidelines.

It is not difficult to imagine that general practitioners may prefer to monitor their own chronic diseases by means of special clinics using nurses and written protocols.

Criteria for managing diseases should be:

- precisely stated
- based on evidence from reviewed research
- prioritized to reflect strength of evidence and influence on outcome
- achievable and measurable
- relevant.

The initial consultation

At the first consultation a doctor should ask himself or herself, what is the diagnosis, how does this fit into the spectrum of this disease, and are there subdivisions of this condition which are of predictive value either for management or prognosis? If this is true, then has this patient been accurately categorized? When was the diagnosis established, and is the patient attending hospital; if so, why, how often and who sees him or her? Finally, what therapeutic goals have been identified and how far have they been achieved? The doctor then has some idea of the problem to be faced and should now ask, 'How do I measure my success in achieving these goals, what do I need to record to do this and in what form should these records be made? What are the likely problems which will arise for this patient and how shall I detect them?'

Subsequent consultations

The following key questions should be asked in any follow-up consultation:

1. When was this case last fully reviewed?
2. When is the next review due?
3. What is the purpose of this consultation?
4. How well does the patient understand the condition?
5. What questions should I now ask?
6. What measurements should be made?
7. What are the indications for me to alter my management?
8. If a change is required, what is to be altered and by how much?
9. When do I need to see this patient again?
10. If the patient fails to return, how shall I be made aware of this fact?

ULCERATIVE COLITIS AND CROHN'S DISEASE

Ulcerative colitis and Crohn's disease will now be used to illustrate the application of some of these principles. The two conditions are considered together because they often overlap; neither is fully understood and they present very similar problems for the general practitioner.

The average general practitioner may expect to have about five cases of Crohn's disease or ulcerative colitis diagnosed amongst his or her patients. As these are chronic diseases the prevalence is considerably more important than the incidence, but one new case of each may be expected every 3 or 4 years.

Crohn's disease

Crohn's disease usually presents with a history of pain suggesting small intestinal colic and mild diarrhoea; sometimes the stools contain blood and mucus or pus. Most cases have low-grade fever and moderate anaemia. The cardinal physical sign is a tender mass in the right lower quadrant. This condition tends to lead a long debilitating course with frequent relapses.

Ulcerative colitis

Ulcerative colitis is a condition in which the colon is inflamed. The onset is insidious and it is characterized by attacks of pain and diarrhoea with blood, mucus and pus. There may be variable fever, loss of weight and anaemia. One in 10 patients suffering from ulcerative colitis has chronic ill health, but 80% are in remission at any one time. Consulting rates for this condition are 0.75 attendances per patient per year.

While Crohn's disease is an intermittent lesion of the small intestine, ulcerative colitis is a continuous lesion of the large intestine. Table 32.1 shows how similar these conditions can be clinically and contrasts them with ischaemic colitis, which is a feature in the older patient.

In applying our principles to these conditions we must answer the questions which have been posed:

- Which diagnosis has been made?
- Has Crohn's disease been clearly differentiated from ulcerative colitis or is there still some doubt?

Crohn's disease has different complications and different implications for the patient, although many difficulties are common to both conditions.

In either case, how active is the disease, has there been a single episode or have there been recurrent attacks? Alternatively, is there an unremitting picture of chronic ill health?

What subdivisions of the condition have predictive value? Clearly it is important to know whether the disease is active or in remission. As we have seen, ulcerative colitis has an 80% remission rate at any one time. The time-scale is also important because the risk of carcinoma in ulcerative colitis increases with the length of time the disease has been present.

Has surgery been undertaken, how long ago, and if not is there any possibility of it being considered in the future?

This not only has an effect on the presence of symptoms but also increases the chances of the emergence of malabsorption.

Is the patient still attending hospital; if so, how often, whom is he or she seeing and what examinations are being made?

The question of routine investigations such as biopsy, colonoscopy and X-ray studies are very relevant to the management of these conditions.

A general practitioner should have the following objectives:

1. to observe the patients who are in remission, seeking evidence of complications

Table 32.1 Diagnosis—ulcerative colitis, Crohn's disease and ischaemic colitis

	Ulcerative colitis	Crohn's disease	Ischaemic colitis
Age (years)	20–40	30–50	50
Symptoms			
1. Blood	Very common	Unusual	Very common
2. Pain	None	Common	Very common
Signs			
1. Tenderness	None	Sometimes	Very common
2. Abdominal mass	None	Sometimes	May develop in next few weeks
3. Anal lesions	Rarely, secondary to infection	Common, often painless, may precede bowel disease	None
Sigmoidoscopy			
1. Rectal involvement	95%	50%	?1%
2. Appearance	Uniform hyperaemia and granulation	Discoloration, oedema, occasional ulceration	Very rare
Radiology	Continuous with rectum	Discontinuous	Left colon especially around splenic flexure
Internal fistulae	None	Sometimes	None
Strictures	Carcinomatous only	Common	Lengthy
Mucosal	Shallow ulcer, granulating polyps	Fissuring ulcer, 'cobblestones'	Mucosal oedema, 'thumb printing'
Clinical presentation	Diarrhoea and rectal bleeding	Very variable, failure to thrive, steatorrhoea	

Reproduced from Beck E R, Francis J L, Souhami R L 1982 *Tutorials in differential diagnosis*, 2nd edn. Pitman Books, London, by permission of the authors.

2. to refer patients to hospital who are experiencing an acute exacerbation
3. to refer for further investigation anyone suspected of having developed complications.

Work is available which provides a comprehensive list of features in the history, examination and investigation of inflammatory bowel disorders which correlate with the diagnosis of Crohn's disease or ulcerative colitis. These features have been given a numerical value and scores obtained by using items on the list have an 85% correlation with the confirmed diagnosis. The list and values are given in Appendix C. A score of more than +5 is thoroughly suggestive of Crohn's disease, and equally a score of less than +5 is predictive of ulcerative colitis. The list must be used with caution because it does not exclude tuberculosis of the bowel and other rare differential diagnoses, but for practical purposes in the UK it is of great value. A general practitioner may score the

patient and make some comparisons over time. The list also provides the questions which should be asked when assessing the present state of either condition. In addition to this the appropriate examination is indicated and some useful information given about the value of blood tests in monitoring the patient's present state. The questions, examinations and tests which should be considered at each consultation are given in Box 32.2.

Table 32.2 shows the possible complications for both diseases and ways in which they might be detected. This is rather a long catalogue but useful as a check-list. The surveillance of these conditions can

---

Box 32.2 Check-list for use at each consultation

When was the patient last reviewed?

When is the next review?

What is his present state?
a. Is he in remission?
b. Is this a subacute attack?
c. Is this an acute attack?

What questions shall I ask?
1. General health
2. Appetite
3. Pain:
   a. Site of
   b. Characteristics
4. Bowels:
   a. Frequency
   b. Presence of blood
   c. Presence of mucus

Examination
1. General appearance—pallor, loss of weight, etc.
2. Abdominal tenderness:
   a. Site
   b. Distension
   c. Masses

Table 32.2 Complications of ulcerative colitis (UC) and Crohn's disease

Type	Specifically	UC	Crohn's	Test
Nutritional	Anaemia	+	+	Hb < 10 g
	Vitamin deficiency	+	+	Various
	Dehydration	+	+	
	Potassium loss	+	+	Serum K
	Protein loss	+	+	Serum albumen < 5 g
Bowel	Toxic dilatation	+		
	Perforation	+	+	
	Bleeding	+	+	Stool for occult blood PR
	Abscesses	+	+	T° WBC > 20 000
	Carcinoma	+		
	Stricture	+	+	
	Small bowel obstruction		+	
	Fistulae		Anal, vagina bladder	Barium studies
Ectoderm	Mouth ulcers	+	+	Examination
	Clubbing	+	+	Examination
	Rashes	+	+	Examination
	Ectopic Crohn's		+	Examination
Arthritis	Various sites	+	+	Ex. X-ray
Ocular	Uveitis, etc.	+	+	Ophthalmoscopy
Hepatic	Various	+	Less common	LFTs
Renal	Calculi	+	+	IVP
	Pyelonephritis	+	+	Test urine. Alb
Thrombophlebitis		+		Examination
Iatrogenic	Drugs	+	+	Various
	Transfusion	+	+	Hb. X-ray
	Surgery	+	+	etc.

Diagnosis				Date of Birth			
Date				Family History			
Hospital/Consultant				Past History			
				Complications			

Date	Pain Site/Type	Bowels			Examination				
		Freq.	Bl.	Muc.	Tend. site. Distension. Mass.	Wt.	T°	Hb° WBC	Other tests- Hosp. review - Next visit etc.

Action points for this patient:-

e.g. Wt loss 7 lbs. Hb < 10 G. Presence of blood in the stool.

WBC > 20,000. Serum albumen < 5G.

32.1 Flow chart for ulcerative colitis.

be made much more explicit by adding a flow chart to the notes. This can be used to record, in a readily accessible manner, successive measurements and symptoms in a way which demonstrates change. It is useful to have action points identified in advance so that patients may be prepared for hospital referral or other new investigations (Fig. 32.1).

The care of chronic disease is one of the emerging challenges to the general practitioner of the future. The ever-advancing frontiers of medicine mean that it is difficult to be sure that each patient is receiving the best available care. The general practitioner should always be questioning himself or herself about the patient, the problem, what is known about the disease, what his or her own knowledge of the condition is and whether there are any signs of change. 'Do I know what to look for and what do I do when I find it?' should always be in the doctor's mind. That is why

this chapter is mostly about asking questions. If they are asked, some of the answers may emerge.

TEACHING POINTS

1. The management of chronic degenerative disease is becoming an increasing part of general practitioners' work.
2. We should always question our management of chronic disease.
3. A flow chart can be valuable for ensuring that routine observations are recorded.
4. Ulcerative colitis and Crohn's disease, although rare, present problems in management.
5. We should be able to detect exacerbations and make appropriate referrals to hospital.
6. There are now published guidelines: get to know them.

33 ALCOHOL ABUSE

Alcoholism is not easy to define and attempting a definition is not very useful. In practical terms alcohol becomes a problem when it interferes with a patient's efficient functioning. Alcohol use is associated with raised morbidity and mortality, the risk rising with increased consumption.

Twenty-eight per cent of men and 11% of women drink more than is recommended. Simple screening instruments are available for detecting people who drink more than this. Brief interventions consisting of assessing the alcohol intake and providing information and advice are effective in reducing alcohol consumption by 20% but the effect on health status is still unclear. Every adult should have an alcohol consumption history taken, using units of alcohol. Advise patients to restrict their drinking to within the recommended levels. Evidence from clinical trials suggests brief interventions are as effective as more expensive specialist treatments. The Health of the Nation campaign and Health Promotion Clinics in primary care provide suitable opportunities to implement these findings. (Source: *Alcohol interventions in primary care*. 1997 Leicestershire NHS Drug and Alcohol Services.)

The current recommended limits for safe drinking are, for men, up to 21 units per week and, for women, 14 units per week (Table 33.1). Excessive drinkers frequently go unnoticed until disaster strikes.

The prevalence of alcoholism is also hard to assess. The most commonly quoted estimate is that there are at least 700 000 problem drinkers in England and Wales, and it has been estimated that a practice of 2500 patients will have a minimum of about 25 alcoholics; but estimates vary widely, and many have been higher than this. The problem is larger than that, however, for alcoholics have families and relatives who often bear the brunt of their problems, with multiplication of the suffering. It is often a hidden problem. It used to be said that a family practitioner knew only 1 in 10 of the alcoholics in his or her practice. Although more recent studies have revised this figure, still considerably less than half the alcoholics will be known to their general practitioner.

The alcoholic may present to the family doctor in a variety of ways, whether it be with marital or employment problems (both common presentations), mental illness or physical disease, e.g. gastritis or a peptic ulcer. The presentation may be even more subtle, e.g. with morning nausea or 'dizzy spells'. It is only infrequently that a patient directly asks for help, so that the doctor must always be alert to the possibility of alcohol playing a part, if not a major part, in a particular patient's problem. The image of the 'Skid Row' alcoholic should not overshadow one's thoughts—they form a tiny part of the problem, and the alcoholic could just as well have been the depressed housewife you have just seen. More often it will be the family and relatives of a patient who will seek your help.

Since general practitioners are in a unique position to diagnose and help patients with an alcohol problem through their knowledge of both patient and family, they should have a reasonable knowledge of the presentations, consequences and warning signs of a deteriorating drinking problem in a patient, together with the help available.

Sylvia Berrington was 45-years-old, a well-dressed and well-spoken married woman living in a large detached house with two grown-up children. She came to the surgery with a specific request for a

Table 33.1 Risk levels and alcohol consumption

Risk	Units per week	
	Women	Men
Low	Up to 14	Up to 21
Increased	15–35	21–50
High	Above 36	Above 51

tranquillizer. I tactfully enquired if there were any particular problems that worried her at present, and she replied that there were 'a few problems at home' but seemed loath to enlarge on this and waited anxiously for the prescription. Further conversation revealed little and I prescribed a 5-day course of chlordiazepoxide, asking her to return then for a further talk. She hurriedly left the surgery. Thus ended a very unsatisfactory consultation. There was nothing in her notes to suggest any underlying problems. Three days later, to my surprise, she came back to the surgery and this time was in a tearful and very unhappy state. Unlike the first consultation, she clearly wanted to talk. 'I'm thinking of leaving my husband,' she cried. Her husband Harold was a successful businessman and the higher he had climbed in his career, the further apart they had grown, and in particular he had started drinking heavily. He had always liked a drink, but drink was now becoming a severe problem and he had been violent towards his wife on several occasions as a result. Alcohol was one of many problems in their relationship, and at the end of the conversation I still had a lot to learn and hoped that she would come back to the surgery with her husband as I had suggested.

In this case it is the wife of the alcoholic who presents. Is this a common presentation?

In a survey of the ways in which alcoholics present in practice, Hore & Wilkins (1976) found that marital complications were the most common presenting problems and this is a typical example. There are many ways in which an alcoholic can present to the doctor and a knowledge of these ways will enable the family practitioner to make the diagnosis more often. Box 33.1 highlights the main areas of life affected by alcoholism and the presentations that may occur in each area. More commonly the patient presents with problems in all areas, e.g. a recently divorced man with financial problems who has lost his job due to repeated absenteeism and presents to you with a severe gastritis.

With the aid of a knowledge of these factors it is a good educational exercise to draw up your own 'at risk' table such as Table 33.2. Another useful exercise would be to devise a scheme for screening for alcoholism within your own practice. Note that recording a suspicion of alcoholism in the notes is essential to alert any other doctor who may see the patient.

Box 33.1 Problems with alcohol

Comment
Male: female ratio 3:1 but falling. Remember the housewife and also the elderly. Especially common in the single, separated and divorced

1. The patient's marriage — Battered wives / Divorce / Marital disharmony / Sexual problems

Comment
It may well be the partner who consults you for 'nerves' or 'depression'. The marriage partner can hardly not be affected

2. The patient at home — Children at risk of developing alcoholism later / Children may present with behaviour problems, delinquency / Child abuse closely correlated with alcoholism / Financial problems / Housing problems / Accidents at home

Comment
There is often a family history of alcoholism. Once again it is emphasized that in treating an alcoholic you are treating the family

3. The patient and the law — Traffic offences including drunken driving / Traffic accidents / Other criminal offences

4. The patient at work — Unemployment / Many job changes / Absenteeism / Accidents at work

Occupations associated with alcoholism — Publicans / Seamen / Barmen / Fishermen

Box 33.1 Problems with alcohol (*contd*)

Hoteliers
Financiers
Cooks
also Doctors!

Comment
Repeated requests for short-term sickness
certification for vague illness is one of the
more common presentations of the alcoholic to
the general practitioner. Such is the cost to
industry that in the United States there are
industrial alcoholism programmes

5. The patient's mental health — Suicide or attempted
suicide
Drug abuse
Wide variety of mental
syndromes, e.g.
delirium,
hallucinations,
dementia, amnesia,
Korsakoff's syndrome
All forms of mood
disturbance
Depression and anxiety
General deterioration
in ability to cope

Comment
Among the most common presentations of the
'hidden alcoholic' are requests for help
because of 'bad nerves' or 'depression'; help
with the alcoholism or underlying social
problem is more appropriate than tranquillizers
and antidepressants. Often the only sign of
alcoholism is a deterioration in appearance or
performance: a businessman with egg on his tie
or an untidy house in the home of a previously
house-proud housewife. Suicide may be a real
risk

6. The patient's physical health — *Major disease*
Cirrhosis of the liver
Alcoholic hepatitis
Anaemia
Peripheral neuritis
Myocardial disease
Peptic ulceration

Box 33.1 Problems with alcohol (*contd*)

Neurological
problems
including fits
Pancreatitis
Obesity
Mallory–Weiss
tears after vomiting
Minor illness
Nausea especially
in the morning
Anorexia
Vomiting
Malnutrition
Tremor
Muscle cramps
Repeated infections
Gastritis

Comment
The most common are the minor ailments,
especially in the morning; thus morning nausea
with a request for time off work might be a
typical consultation highly suggestive of
alcoholism. It is said that only about 10% of
alcoholics develop permanent liver disease,
although most will have fatty changes

Blood tests
The three most useful are a blood alcohol level
(especially if raised in the morning), the
gamma glutamyl transpeptidase (raised in most
alcoholics), and an unexplained macrocytosis
in the blood film

Physical examination
Waiting for the classical signs of liver damage
as a result of the alcoholism is not the way to
practice preventative medicine, but obviously a
patient presenting *de novo* with spider naevi,
palmar erythema, clubbing, etc. must be
investigated. The swollen ruddy complexion of
the face in an overweight patient is one of my
triggers of suspicion. A tremor is a sign to note

*Mr and Mrs Berrington did come to the surgery
together. They had discussed some of their marital
problems and for the first time Harold had accepted
that he had a drinking problem.*

Table 33.2 At risk of alcoholism

At risk: suspect drink	Alcoholism very likely	Alcoholism virtually certain
Gastritis, anorexia, fatigue, peripheral neuropathy, etc.	Smells of alcohol in surgery	Asks for help
Flushed face	Spouse complains	Cirrhosis
Morning symptoms (especially Monday morning)	High blood alcohol when taken in the morning	Withdrawal symptoms
Marital problems and sexual problems	Repeated injury to spouse	Classical physical or psychological sequelae
Work problems including absenteeism	Deranged liver function tests in	Intoxicated at time of presentation
Depression/anxiety	absence of obvious cause	
Attempted suicide		
Problems with child neglect		
History of blackouts, insomnia		
Tremor		
Problems with the law		
Occupation at risk (see Box 33.1)		

In talking to him, how would you assess the severity of the problem?

As shown in Box 33.1, alcohol affects all areas of a patient's life and can rarely be contained in one area. One of the greatest assets a family doctor can possess is the art of tactful and relaxed but inquiring conversation. The areas can be explored by friendly open-ended questions to build up the picture. Select a few of the more important areas. The marital difficulties were talked of at length and I also asked Harold about his work, general health and whether there were any financial problems. I then came round to talking directly of his drinking. A 'drinking history' of such patients should be taken—a less familiar pattern of history-taking to many doctors.

The quantity, type and time of drinking is of obvious importance. The previous 7 days consumption should be regarded as the best guide to average consumption. There are also a series of questions useful in deciding if a drinking problem is getting out of control. These are not to be asked as a list but can usually be brought into the conversation. The questions are sometimes seen as threatening by the patient but need not be, and once a few have been answered affirmatively there is little point in proceeding. I find their use more of a reminder of which areas to explore in a drinking history rather than as a specific list of questions to be asked. Some questions serving to indicate a deteriorating drinking problem getting out of control are these:

- Do you lose time at work because of drink?

- Is your job at risk due to drink?
- Are you less efficient in your daily routine due to drink?
- Have you had financial problems due to drink?
- Do you crave for drink at a particular time of day?
- Does drink cause you to have difficulty sleeping?
- Do you drink to forget your problems?
- Do you drink to build up confidence?
- Do you drink alone?
- Do you want a drink the next morning?
- Have you ever lost your memory or 'blacked out' due to drink?

Ask particularly of drinking and symptoms experienced in the morning. There are useful self-assessment questionnaires.

Physical examination of the chronic alcoholic may reveal the ravages of alcohol, but by the time the signs are present the history has been a long one and the alcoholic is probably well known to the doctor. This is not, however, always the case and I have seen a patient present with advanced cirrhosis who never visited the doctor and denied drinking (a fact not substantiated by the wife). This patient had no physical symptoms and I did not examine him at this visit. For the occasional suspected alcoholic who denies drink one might consider a blood test to look for macrocytosis in the blood film, a raised blood alcohol level and a raised gamma glutamyl transpeptidase—this last test is particularly useful.

During the course of several consultations I discovered that Harold Berrington had a far more serious alcohol problem than I had at first guessed. He was drinking in the morning and arranging his appointments around what amounted to a 'schedule' of alcohol consumption; more particularly the business was beginning to suffer. He was at first reluctant to ask for help but was anxious to stem further marital disharmony, and after a few further talks he himself came alone to the surgery with a positive manner asking what help was available.

How would you guide him?

The very fact that he realizes he has a problem and wishes to overcome it is a most optimistic start to alleviating his drinking. One of the major steps in combating an alcohol problem is the acceptance by the patient that he has indeed a problem and may need help for it. Another good prognostic feature in this case was the presence of his interested wife, who was as keen as he was to tackle the problem and proved to be very supportive. The husband was lucky on another count too, having no financial problems, an excellent job and a good home. Without these features the prognosis is less favourable for any given patient.

How then should a family doctor approach a patient with an alcohol problem, once it is recognized? The seven stages gone through in a typical case are as outlined below.

Stage 1: Analysis of the problem once discovered

- How long has there been any problem?
- Why is the patient presenting at this place and time?
- Are there any reasons for the alcoholism or for this acute episode?
- What areas of life are affected, especially the family?
- What is the patient's mental state and attitude?
- Is alcohol affecting the patient's physical state?
- Is the patient's work suffering?
- Establish some form of drinking history.

We have dealt with some of these in the case history but note that we have said nothing of causative factors. The family doctor is in a unique position to determine causative factors, and no help or treatment is likely to be successful without a knowledge of the reasons why a patient is consuming too much or becoming addicted to alcohol. Similarly a crisis event (divorce, loss of

job, etc.) may turn a moderate drinker into a problem one. In this case there were a multitude of factors—marital problems played a part and business pressures too, but what surprised me most was the insight I obtained into the patient's character. He proved to be far from the ruthless, aggressive and dynamic businessman he portrayed and he was really quite insecure inside and held a low opinion of himself. He also revealed that he felt unable to cope successfully with the increasing competitiveness within his business, but dared not mention this to his wife as he thought she would lose respect for him. All this serves to illustrate one thing—if you have time and can talk about such problems you may well uncover a great deal. The groundwork is so vital; if you cannot uncover the roots of a problem, success will be limited and relapse rate high.

The role of tests

The following tests have some part to play in the assessment of the effects of alcohol. In doubtful cases we are using blood alcohol levels in practice and they reveal some surprising results!

- The gamma glutamyl transpeptidase (γGT) test reflects drinking in the last few days and, if raised, can take about 3 weeks to subside. This test can be used to assess recent alcohol consumption
- Mean corpuscular volume (MCV) reflects longer term drinking. The average life of a red cell is 60 days so the MCV is increased by the toxic effect of alcohol on the bone marrow. This test can be used to assess longer term alcohol consumption.

It should, however, be remembered that only 65% of in-patient alcoholics have one or both of these tests abnormal.

Stage 2: Acceptance by the patient of the problem

This patient accepted that the problem existed. This is a key task for the family doctor.

Stage 3: Maintaining motivation

A patient must be motivated to help himself; the strength of this motivation will vary from patient to patient and the source of the motivation will vary. For this patient, preservation of his marriage and improvement in his business were obvious motivations. Stress these benefits to the patient and list all the areas which may benefit, not least the patient's health. Remind the patient that alcohol is an addictive drug.

Stage 4: Involving the family

The hardest to help are often those who are alone. Good family support goes a long way in treatment. I had several talks with this couple and it became apparent that they had not really been communicating for some time; in particular, the wife became aware of the severity of the business pressures on her husband. If you find yourself out of your depth, do not be afraid to refer for marital counselling or to the Alcohol Team.

Stage 5: Positive help; the first steps to controlling drinking

Having established the problems and a positive attitude, how can the doctor help further? Often by this stage the patient has already been helped substantially by coming to realize the problems and may require little else but some advice. Brief advice together with an educational leaflet can be very effective at reducing alcohol consumption and may reduce the number of problem drinkers in a practice by up to 50%.

Multidisciplinary teams should be able to provide rapid assessment and treatment. Alcohol withdrawal is usually the first step and the patient with dependency who 'just wants to cut down' must be firmly encouraged to stop altogether, for some months at least. Withdrawal can occur at high levels of alcohol because of the tolerance that develops in the liver enzymes. Few drinkers connect their early morning anxiety or irritable wakening, depression, night sweats, diarrhoea or the narrowing of their life style with alcohol and one of the reasons for abstinence is to demonstrate improvement in these symptoms, making future management more likely to succeed.

There has been a great deal of controversy over whether one should aim for total abstinence or 'controlled drinking'. The answer is probably that it depends on the patient. There are severe alcoholics who are chronically dependent who may need withdrawal in hospital and experience severe withdrawal symptoms. In the majority of patients you will meet, supervision by family and doctor (and/or other members of the health care team) can achieve some measure of withdrawal at home and a pattern of controlled

drinking established. For most with a drinking problem I would counsel a controlled drinking approach, but with certain alcoholics, notably severely dependent alcoholics, those with medical problems, e.g. cirrhosis, pancreatitis, etc., and those for whom lessening drink has previously failed, abstinence is the better aim. This patient made me realize that in his business abstinence was very difficult as he was often entertaining clients.

The initial help may involve four areas:

a. *Detoxification.* Detoxification at home is preferable. Alcohol withdrawal can be managed at home in most patients, but not in the severely dependent and addicted, who are best admitted to hospital. Much is made of withdrawal symptoms but in practice few problems are encountered, especially in the mild to moderate alcoholics you are managing at home. Some time off work may help some, as may a short prescription for chlormethiazole (Heminevrin) or a benzodiazepine. The chlormethiazole is started at a high dose and tailed off. Much has also been made of vitamin B deficiency, but this is again the problem largely of the severe addict.

b. *Help with other problems.* We have said that alcohol problems do not occur in isolation and that we wish to help tackle all areas if possible.
Consider: (i) Marriage guidance counselling
(ii) Help with financial problems, housing problems, etc.
(iii) Sexual counselling
(iv) Careers counselling, retraining, etc.

These problems will involve the doctor in asking colleagues (social worker, health visitor, etc.) for help.

c. *The patient's physical and mental health.* Some conditions may need referral, e.g. for gastroscopy if recurrent epigastric pain is experienced. Be particularly aware of mental problems; depression may need to be treated skilfully, and above all beware the risk of suicide. If there is a suicidal element the patient may best be referred.

d. *Advice* (see below). My patient coped with his withdrawal period well. I made a contract with him to control his drinking and the advice I gave him to help was this:

(i) Remember, alcohol is a drug of addiction.
(ii) Keep a diary of how much you drink.
(iii) Try to drink beverages with the least alcohol

content: (glass of wine = single whisky = glass of sherry = 1/2 pint of beer).
(iv) Define absolute limits for consumption, e.g. the equivalent of 2 pints of beer a day at first.
(v) Don't drink alone.
(vi) Try to eat something when drinking.
(vii) Drink slowly, never gulping.

When he came back to see me a few weeks later he showed me his diary and things had indeed improved, and this was verified by his wife. If controlled drinking fails then abstinence is generally advised and further referral may be necessary.

Relaxation training is helpful and an increasing number of general practitioners are learning how to use these techniques.

Stage 6: Is referral necessary, and where to?

There have been several attempts to compare different treatments and approaches to the management of alcoholism and the results have been disappointing; no treatment approach as yet has emerged as noticeably superior to others, although behaviour psychotherapy seems to be effective in many cases (Smith *BMJ* October 1981).

Types of treatment include:

- Psychotherapy—individual, group, family therapy
- Alcoholics Anonymous—in effect group therapy
- Out-patient care
- Hospital in-patient care
- Community care—day centres, home visiting, community alcohol team
- Aversion therapy
- Behaviour therapy, including social skills training
- Use of specific drugs, e.g. disulfiram (Antabuse), which may be effective for well-motivated but impulsive drinkers, and acamprosate, a new GABA antagonist useful in maintaining abstinence in alcohol-dependent patients.

The family doctor will know what facilities for help are available in the area. For example, in Leicester we are fortunate in having a Community Alcohol Treatment Team of a consultant psychiatrist, social worker, community psychiatric nurse, etc. There is also a day centre and an Alcohol Advice Centre. They visit at home and try vigorously to follow-up patients. Examples of local services available are listed in Box 33.2.

> **Box 33.2** Local services available
>
> National Health Service Community Drug and Alcohol Service
> Mental Health Service Unit
> Community Alcohol Team
> Community Drug Team
> Residential Hostels
> Action for Youth Trust
> Drug and Alcohol Help Line
> Local Alcohol Advice Team for dissemination of information
> Local Alcohol Advice Centre
>
> This list is based on local arrangements but there are equivalent services throughout the country. It is advisable to keep a list of local telephone numbers

Alcoholics Anonymous (AA) groups exist in most areas. They do not suit everyone, but many people have been helped by them and nothing is lost by going to a meeting. By being involved in AA activities and talking about their problems in this way some alcoholics do achieve abstinence (note that abstinence rather than controlled drinking is the aim of AA).

Referral for psychotherapy and behaviour therapy is useful for some patients. The results achieved depend heavily on the therapist.

The use of Antabuse requires considerable willpower and occasionally produces severe reactions; it is thus not particularly appropriate to the family doctor, nor is aversion therapy, which is much less popular now.

A main area of referral is for psychiatric help for patients with severe personality problems or psychiatric disease, either as the cause or the result of alcoholism. Many of these problems are very resistant to treatment. One fruitful area, though, is with the shy, confidence-lacking patient needing social skills training and help in boosting his confidence in himself.

Hospital in-patient care may be required for the severe alcoholic.

Harold and his wife proved to be an involved case, as many are. The husband's drinking problem improved, largely due to the continued support of his wife, and there was an improvement in their marriage, partly because of the wife's increasing understanding of the husband's work. His business took a turn for the better. He did not need a referral.

Stage 7: Follow-up

All doctors should maintain an interest in their alcoholics; alcoholism is just as much a chronic disease for follow-up as is, say, hypertension. Continuity of care is the family doctor's role.

The outlook for the alcoholic is not as dismal as many doctors suppose. About one in three can be cured of the problem, another third can be substantially helped, and only one-third derive little benefit from our activities.

Summarize the role of the family physician in the management of alcoholism.

Box 33.3 lists the main roles of the family doctor in

Box 33.3 Role of the family practitioner in alcoholism

1. Health education in the surgery, lecturing, the media, etc.
2. Diagnosis. Screening
3. Helping the individual once diagnosed:
   a. assessment
   b. treatment, including the family and involving other team members
   c. referral if appropriate
   d. follow-up
4. Research
5. As a member of professional organizations to press for government help and to determine government policy

---

cases of alcoholism. Not much has been said of health education and prevention of alcoholism, but that is a different story.

In order to manage alcoholism effectively the family doctor must have a sympathetic approach, a knowledge of alcoholism and its management, a good support team and a detailed knowledge of the local facilities in the area in which he or she practises.

TEACHING POINTS

1. The general practitioner will know less than half the alcoholics in his or her practice.
2. Have a high index of suspicion and learn the ways in which alcoholics can present to their general practitioner. If you suspect alcoholism record it in the notes.
3. Among common presentations remember marital problems, repeated requests for sickness certification, minor symptoms (especially in the morning) and depression.
4. The key to treatment lies in the patient's acceptance that he or she has a problem.
5. Involve the family as much as possible.
6. List the 'seven stages approach' outlined in this chapter.
7. Remember that alcoholism, like hypertension, is a problem requiring long-term follow-up.
8. Know the facilities in your area which may help a given alcoholic in your practice.
9. Every adult should have an alcohol consumption history taken, using units of alcohol.
10. Advise patients to restrict their drinking to within the recommended levels.
11. Reduction in alcohol consumption can be achieved by using simple advice (25–35%).

34 OUR FAVOURITE TUTORIAL: A DIFFICULT PATIENT

Every now and then you meet what can only be described as a difficult patient. A frequent attender presents with problems fitting no known diagnosis and conspicuously fails to respond to any of the various treatments, which have been offered in hope rather than expectation. Any general practitioner will immediately recognise these most difficult of patients. So it was one Thursday morning in April when I met David for the first time.

David was a 42-year-old unemployed car mechanic. He was married and lived on a council estate near the surgery. He was a frequent attender, usually seeing one of the partners for a few months before moving on to another. His notes were voluminous and filled with letters from his previous hospital referrals and included many ECGs. I glanced through his notes before he came in. There was little of interest on the summary card apart from vague references to 'anxiety', 'possible angina', 'cardiac neurosis' and 'myocardial ischaemia—unproven'. The letters were more helpful—he had clearly been extensively investigated for chest pain but with nothing found. He had had at least two exercise tests and an embarrassing number of normal ECGs. His notes recorded many examinations of the heart, blood pressure, etc., the diagnosis usually ending up as one of 'anxiety'. He had been on and off diazepam frequently in the past.

As David entered he coughed nervously. He looked worried, avoided eye contact and played with his hands nervously while he talked. His problem was that his heart seemed to be missing beats every now and then and, since he was prone to chest pain anyway, he thought he ought to see a doctor. My heart sank. It seemed all too clear that once again David was moving towards either a cardiac examination, ECG and perhaps hospital referral and/or a prescription for a beta-blocker.

Where should I start? I did indeed give David a thorough examination and, apart from a tachycardia of 100, could find nothing. I reassured him that all appeared to be well but this fell on stony ground. 'Why does my heart miss a beat then doctor?' he asked. I explained this may well be normal and desperately searched through his notes, triumphantly producing a normal ECG from a few months before, but to no avail—'My heart didn't miss beats then doctor.' I was cornered—perhaps I was missing something? Could he be thyrotoxic? What about a 24-hour ECG recording? Is it just anxiety? I resolved to do a blood test for possible hyperthyroidism and see him again in a few days, earlier if any further symptoms developed. Thus ended a most unsatisfactory consultation—I felt totally deflated and David left the surgery as worried as when he had entered. His return in a few days was, in fact, equally unsatisfactory—his heart was still missing beats, the result of the blood test wasn't, of course, back yet and the examination was still normal. I was completely undecided what to do, he had seen every cardiologist within 20 miles and an occasional psychiatrist too. His ECGs already needed a separate packet! It was nearing my Friday afternoon tutorial so I hoped that my trainer would come to the rescue.

The tutorial

My trainer had a broad and knowing smile when I presented David's case. He knew David well, as indeed did all the partners. The tutorial took place in several stages, as outlined below.

What were my difficulties with this consultation?

We began the tutorial by looking at my difficulties. My trainer agreed that David was a particularly difficult problem but was pleased we were talking about him, as it raised several important issues. One of my main difficulties was undoubtedly an inability to live with the uncertainty of failing to make a satisfactory diagnosis. This is common with new registrars and tolerating uncertainty is an acquired ability, as my trainer pointed out. All too often you can't make a conventional diagnosis.

My second difficulty was one all new registrars and partners experience—to see as a new patient someone already well known to other partners in the practice. In not already knowing David I was clearly at a major disadvantage but, as my trainer noted, sometimes a fresh face can shed new light on a problem—supposing he did have thyrotoxicosis!

I had few doubts about my clinical acumen with regard to the differential diagnosis of missed heartbeats or about my ability to perform a good cardiological examination. It is, in fact, rare for registrars to have problems of this nature.

I identified a further problem relating to myself (and, I suppose, many other registrars)—a reluctance to diagnose anxiety. Anxiety is not an easy problem to deal with, and when does it require a prescription and for how long should the drugs be prescribed? We discussed this problem.

My trainer furthered the tutorial by suggesting that, as a relatively new registrar, some of my difficulties in approaching this consultation might be due to a lack of experience in communicating with patients like David. More of this later.

What problems do patients like David pose general practitioners?

We briefly went on to look at the problems posed by such frequent attenders as David. How much time should the general practitioner spend with such patients? What expectations of doctors do patients like David have? Would they benefit from seeing one doctor only or should the load be shared? What about communications between hospital doctors and general practitioners with regard to such patients? How might they best be helped? Is the doctor the best person to manage them or are other members of the health care team more appropriate? What does David think about his condition and its management to date?

Critical evaluation of the consultation

My trainer asked several questions about my handling of David. What questions did I ask David about his palpitations? Did I explore his worries further? Why

did he choose to consult the new registrar and not a partner? Why did he come this particular Thursday morning? How did I go about reassuring David? What did David expect from this consultation? As I wrestled with these questions from my trainer, it became apparent that I might not have really understood at all why David had come to see me. What did David want from the consultation? Perhaps all David did want was reassurance about his missing heartbeats, but I began to have nagging doubts that important areas of the consultation had been missed out. It occurred to me that David had presented similarly to this many times before and a plethora of doctors had examined him thoroughly and ordered a blood test or ECG. Perhaps a different approach was warranted. I still, however, couldn't convince myself that I shouldn't perform an ECG.—after all it was a new symptom for David. Perhaps, I pondered, this is merely a reflection of hospital training and would only reinforce to David that something might be wrong.

A strategy for further consultations

My trainer took the lead and began to construct a strategy for the next consultation with David. He suggested we see him together, which we subsequently did. I was determined to have a ECG.

My trainer bet it would be normal (it was!). Having ruled out serious disease, my trainer suggested we adopt the following strategy.

1. We would first confront David with the fact that his symptoms had been extensively investigated and were not pathological.

2. We would enquire of David why he was presenting in this way, at this time. What were his fears? What particularly worried him?

3. We would then explore his fears and anxieties fully (e.g. fear of dying, employment and marital worries).

4. We would never revert to the original symptoms.

5. We would try to put ourselves in David's shoes ('You must feel …').

6. We would, in a kind and sympathetic manner, ask David what he would like us to do, given these are his problems.

7. We would reassure, give practical advice and offer continuing support.

8. We would arrange with David a future consultation to monitor progress.

Follow-up to the tutorial

There were several areas I wished to explore but especially that of the management of anxiety. When should drugs be used and, if drugs were inappropriate, what about relaxation therapy and hypnosis? My trainer directed me to some further reading and mentioned a general practitioner with an interest in hypnotherapy, who might be a useful contact if I wished to take it any further. We also decided that it would be interesting to have a look at the notes of a few other frequent attenders at the surgery and use these as a basis for a future discussion. Were there any common factors in these patients? My enthusiasm was fired! I resolved to follow David as long as I was with the practice.

What I learnt from the tutorial

I learnt a lot from this tutorial. There are no easy answers to problems like David's and every general practitioner develops his or her own way of approaching them. A registrar new to general practice has, however, little experience of patients like David and needs some guidelines. The strategy we devised for David's consultation may not be agreed by all but it as least gave me a starting point. This questioning approach to a consultation—asking many questions rather than continually providing answers—was relatively new to me. I was also surprised in this case by the onus being placed so much with the patient.

Teaching communicating and consulting skills is by no means easy. A registrar will learn most by sitting in with the trainer and the other partners, to some extent mimicking their behaviour. I was particularly pleased, therefore, to see David again with my trainer conducting the consultation (see below).

I shall always remember David with affection. I saw him several times in my registrar year and grew to look forward to our next consultation. I learned a lot about managing anxiety and learnt to tolerate more the uncertainty of not always arriving at a precise and firm diagnosis. Why then was this my favourite tutorial? It was my favourite tutorial quite simply because discussing David opened up a whole new vista for me about looking at the reasons why patients consult and how to deal with situations where you haven't got all the answers! To some extent you can learn much of the clinical side of general practice with some directed effort at appropriate reading, but we spend the whole of our working lives learning how better to communicate with our patients. This tutorial showed me one approach to a difficult consultation. I can't honestly say that I have used the complete strategy since, but I've certainly incorporated parts of it into my style of consultation with a few particular patients. Training is all about improving the ways you talk to and help your patients. I can certainly say that this tutorial helped me to look much more closely at that most common part of our daily work—the consultation.

David came back to see us and my trainer conducted the consultation, sticking closely to our strategy. David's symptoms had resolved and his thyroid function was normal. My trainer had a long and frank discussion with David and David certainly seemed quite relieved at the end, having discussed his fears and worries at great length. He left the surgery a much happier man.

TEACHING POINTS

1. One has to accept that not all consultations can be brought to a satisfactory conclusion.
2. A general practitioner has to tolerate the anxiety of not always arriving at a precise and firm diagnosis.
3. Registrars can learn to handle difficult situations by sitting in with their trainers.

35 FIRST STEPS IN AUDIT

Audit is, in fact, quite a simple concept. It is a process whereby you look critically at an area of care and activity and measure the performance of those providing that care, or undertaking that activity, in relation to what has been agreed to be the ideal standard of care.

Audit is sometimes used synonymously with performance review. In effect, you are seeing how you actually perform compared with a set standard. This is not the end of the audit process: once deficiencies in performance have been identified, a programme of change should be instituted. Finally the whole process (often known as the audit cycle, Fig. 35.1) is completed by reviewing how these changes have improved performance after a suitable time interval—have you achieved (or nearly achieved) your ideal standard? If you are still far short of the standard you will need to identify the reasons, institute change and begin the whole cycle again.

Why undertake audit?

There must be a good reason to do any activity, and compulsion is not one of them. You undertake audit to improve an area of patient care or solve a particular problem for the practice, with resulting benefit for the patients, practice or practice team. The main watchword is improvement: you audit to improve.

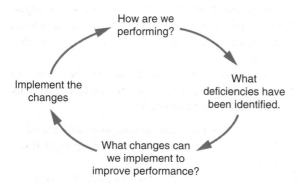

Fig. 35.1 The audit cycle.

Many texts on audit emphasize the secondary value of audit, in terms of professional development and establishing a practice team approach to problem-solving. Audit can be a stimulating intellectual exercise, but it can also be frustrating and very hard work. If you are going to undertake audit, it should be for a specific purpose.

Compulsory audit

There is, however, an element of compulsion to audit. For example, audit is set to be an important component of the summative assessment package. Moreover, all general practitioners, as part of the process of receiving payment for diabetes and asthma care, are required to audit these activities. These audits, together with audits for other health promotion work, take up many bytes of practice computer capacity.

Types of audit

There are four types of audit:

- *Self-audit*: how am I performing in a particular area?
- *Practice-based audit*: how are we, as a practice, performing in a particular area?
- *Peer-group audit*: how are peer groups performing in a particular area?
- *External audit*: Big Brother is watching YOU!

What can I audit?

When deciding what is a suitable subject to audit, it is best to choose an area of care or activity that interests you or that poses a particular problem for you, your practice or your patients. You must consider three elements when choosing a topic:

- Performance—you must measure performance.
- Standard—you need to be measuring against an agreed standard.

- Change—you will be seeking change to improve the status quo.

Almost any area of practice activity can be audited. Five broad areas to consider are clinical practice, practice finance, prescribing, referrals and practice management (Table 35.1).

Seven steps to audit

Undertaking your first audit can be simplified by following the 'Seven Steps to Audit':

1. Choose a suitable topic.
2. Agree your objectives in carrying out the audit.
3. Identify your ideal standards of care.
4. Analyse your current performance.
5. Identify your deficiencies compared with the set standard.
6. Institute change to improve performance.
7. After a time interval, see if the changes have improved performance.

Step 1: Choose an audit

It is important to keep an audit as simple as possible. You should be looking at a clearly defined, narrow area of performance amenable to standard setting and to assessable change. We will take two examples—patients with diagnosed hypothyroidism (clinical practice) and the new registration check (practice management). Both are circumscribed areas of care or activity that are simple to audit. Care of cancer patients or item-of-service payments are clearly much

wider concepts that would be more difficult to audit. Hypothyroidism and new registration checks also fulfil the other criteria for choosing an audit:

- Choose an audit that will benefit patients or the practice.
- Choose an area you are interested in (I'm quite interested in thyroid problems, and practice revenue is always of interest).
- Choose a common problem, enabling you to collect data over a reasonable time interval, e.g. 3 months.
- Choose an area where standards can be agreed, performance measured and changes instituted.
- Choose an area where you will not totally disrupt the practice with folders of forms and protocols for everyone to fill in.

Step 2: Agree your aims and objectives

The audit is likely to be a group activity, so there should be mutually agreed aims and objectives.

The aims of the hypothyroidism audit could be to improve standards of care for patients, ensure that patients on thyroxine have been properly diagnosed, that all patients are reviewed regularly, and that all hypothyroid patients have thyroid-stimulating hormone (TSH) levels in the normal range. The aim of the new registration check audit could be to improve the uptake of these checks, which would considerably enhance practice profitability.

Step 3: Identify your ideal standards of care

The ideal standard of care is that every patient with hypothyroidism has fulfilled your criteria and that every patient has received a new registration check. In practice you may have to substitute 'acceptable' or 'realistically achievable' for the word 'ideal'. While it is ideal that every patient attends for a new registration check within the claimable 3-month period, a more realistic, nearly ideal standard would be that 75% attend.

What standards and criteria can we then draw up for our two audits? The ideal standards for patients with hypothyroidism might be:

- for each patient to have an unequivocally raised TSH (specify the value) before starting thyroxine treatment
- for each patient on thyroxine to have had their TSH measured within the last year

Table 35.1 Areas of general practice which can be audited

Area	Notes
Clinical practice	Diabetes, asthma and hypertension are major areas, but almost any clinical area can be audited
Practice finance	Income areas are particularly popular, e.g. how you are performing on items of service payments like tetanus vaccination or contraceptive claims (as a percentage of the eligible practice population)
Prescribing	Audit can concern itself with wider, perhaps financial, issues or narrower specific areas, e.g. HRT prescription
Referrals	An audit of referral patterns is a relatively simple and painless exercise
Practice management	For example, the appointments system, the visiting system or the computer prescribing system

- for each patient to appear on the practice's register of patients with hypothyroidism
- for the most recent TSH value to fall within a set range (specify the range you feel appropriate).

The ideal standard for the new registration check audit would be for 75% of eligible patients to attend a check within the claimable 3-month period.

In both examples, I have given only a few areas to address. I have kept my audit simple.

Step 4: Analyse your current performance
The next stage is data collection. You must motivate all those participating and make sure that data are efficiently collected, with no errors, observer variation or incomplete record-keeping. Good records are the key to a successful audit.

How and what data you collect (and who collects it) will depend on your audit. With the hypothyroidism audit, the first step is to identify patients on thyroxine (from computer repeat prescriptions), and then analyse their records to determine their TSH at diagnosis, the date of last TSH measurement and its values, and whether the patient is logged into your practice register.

Data collection will always raise challenges, such as patients whose previous results were in terms of thyroxine level not TSH, or patients on thyroxine who are not on repeats, but see the nurse or general practitioner regularly instead. Similarly, could there be newly diagnosed patients who are not yet on the computer? Inevitably, even with such a seemingly simple audit, you will have to chase doctors and records, and may have to adapt your criteria (e.g. include thyroxine in the initial diagnosis criteria).

For the new registration check audit you will need to tally claims and registrations.

Step 5: Identify your deficiencies
You must now look at your performance and compare it with your set standards. You may uncover deficiencies, such as only 50% of patients on thyroxine having had their TSH measured in the last year, or only 40% of patients eligible for a new registration check having actually received one. Any deficiencies need to be discussed at a practice meeting; the reasons for these deficiencies and how they might be addressed should be reviewed.

Step 6: Institute and implement changes
The next stage is crucial—changing and improving your methods, systems and efforts to ensure better results in future. The deficiencies identified by the hypothyroidism audit could lead to you adopting a computerized patient recall system or a tagging system in the notes, and some patients may need to be recalled. With new registration checks you may need a new practice policy, e.g. practice nurses performing the check immediately when patients register, asking patients to return for a check will substantially lower the take-up rate.

Step 7: Have changes improved performance?
After a certain time, you need to evaluate the data to see whether the planned changes have been adhered to and if they have improved performance. This stage is important: it completes the audit cycle and shows if you have been successful in your audit. A decent time interval (e.g. 6–12 months) should be allowed before evaluating the changes.

First, you need to assess if the changes you suggested have been put into operation—is there now an effective recall system for hypothyroid patients, and do all patients have their TSH measured annually? Do the nurses now have opportunistic slots for new registration checks? Finally, after say a year, how many patients still have no TSH values in their notes, and what percentage of new patients now have a new registrations check within the 3-month claimable period?

Final thoughts

As you can see from the above, audit does not necessarily create a heavy workload and it can give tangible, not to mention profitable, results. An improved uptake for new registration checks will generate considerable income for a practice and may also result in claims, e.g. for contraception or tetanus vaccination. It all depends on attitude. When used as a practical problem-solving tool, audit can be a friend, not an enemy.

Acknowledgements
This chapter first appeared as an article in *Training Update* (March 1996) and is reproduced with permission from Reed Healthcare Communications Ltd.

36 THE PROJECT

Within all of us there is a spirit of enquiry, and general practice throws up sufficient questions to satiate even the most active human brain—plenty of topics for a project. But what exactly is a project?

A question of definition

A project is an attempt to answer a question (or questions) by means of collecting data, analysing the information obtained and drawing appropriate conclusions. A project might be a large, multicentre study or the effort of an individual doctor to answer a particular question. A project is not audit—this topical activity has a more precise definition (see Ch. 35).

A question of enthusiasm

Why should a general practice registrar carry out a project at all? Projects should be undertaken for positive reasons, such as:

- to answer a question of particular relevance to the individual or his or her surgery
- for the intellectual stimulus of responding to a challenge
- for the enjoyment and personal fulfilment of a job well done.

A major benefit of project work can be the development of a special and enduring interest in an area of practice. There is tremendous scope for existing and prospective general practitioners to exploit such special areas of expertise or knowledge—general practice research and publication is still in its infancy when compared with the output from hospital specialities. While pursuing your project, you will establish contacts with like-minded general practice researchers, sowing the seeds of professional relationships that should sustain your enthusiasm even in the darkest hours of your working life. Compulsion is the poorest reason for undertaking a project. Project work can be time-intensive, may well be frustrating and is occasionally morale-draining—success is not guaranteed.

A question of choice

How should you select a suitable topic for your project? This question is easy to answer: choose an area in which you are interested. There are only two other major considerations:

- You must be able to collect adequate data to complete the project in a reasonable time (e.g. less than 3 months). Choose common conditions rather than Behçet's syndrome! You need not confine yourself to clinical issues—projects on practice management topics or consultation problems are just as valid.
- You must be able to pose a simple question or questions capable of being answered in the period allowed for your project. Do not question the cause of cancer in your first study.

The planning stage

Planning is the critical stage of project work. A badly designed project is doomed to failure, whereas a well-planned study should run smoothly with the minimum of exertion or stress. About one-third of the total project time should be spent on the planning (Box 36.1), which can be broken down into six tasks (Box 36.2).

Define the aims of your project

Pose a simple question or questions, e.g. how many women consult the practice with cystitis during a 3-month period, and in how many of these cases does culture of a mid-stream urine specimen (MSU) show a significant bacterial growth?

Decide on an end-point

Just as all projects should have a starting date, all should have an end-point. In the cystitis example, the

Box 36.1 When planning your first project, keep it simple

1. Ask an easy question, e.g. why do patients attend for HRT?
2. Use a simple method to gather information, e.g. distribute a questionnaire to those attending for HRT
3. Choose a common condition so that you will collect enough data in time

This simple project could also be expanded to look at different aspects of HRT consultation and prescribing: what do patients expect from HRT, how long do they expect to continue taking it, do they check their breasts regularly, etc? As with all projects, the first question will generate as many questions for future projects as answers to the question posed

Box 36.2 Allow one-third of the total project time for planning

1. Define the aims of your project
2. Decide on an end-point
3. Undertake background reading
4. Subject your plan to peer review
5. Construct your protocol
6. Motivate all those participating in the project

end-point would be time-related (3 months). In the HRT example (Box 36.1), the end-point would be related to the number of patients—you might choose to question 50 patients, for example. Fixing an end-point at the outset is essential; it is not permissible to start a study with no fixed end-point and conclude it when you have recruited an interesting patient.

Undertake background reading

You must acquaint yourself with current publications on your chosen subject. A short literature search will provide you with some general answers, although these will not relate to your particular practice population. Studying some articles on the subject will help you refine your questions and perhaps suggest additions and alternatives.

Subject your plan to peer review

Before constructing your protocol, discuss your ideas with someone with research and project experience; their suggestions will probably save embarrassment later on. Local university lecturers or general practice tutors could be the first point of call. In every locality there will be general practitioners who have relevant experience or can direct you to someone who has. Ask the contact to criticize your final protocol.

Construct your protocol

Study design is a complex area, but there are three golden rules to observe.

1. Standardize. For a project to have any meaning at all, there must be standardization. For the cystitis project, you must define exactly what you mean by cystitis or a 'significant growth'. In the HRT example, your definition of a 'patient attending for HRT' must be crystal clear. Are these to be new patients starting HRT, those already on HRT and attending for follow-up, those just requesting advice on HRT, or all three groups? If you decide to include all three groups, how are you going to identify to which group a patient belongs? Every patient in a study must receive exactly the same questionnaire/advice/tests/treatment under exactly the same conditions. Entry criteria (defining which patients will be entered into the study) must be fully standardized and adhered to, with every patient entering the study fulfilling exactly the same criteria. If you are tempted to bend the rules—allowing a patient to enter the study who does not quite fit the criteria but will make up the numbers—the value is lost.

2. Design any questionnaire with care. Many studies founder as a result of poor questionnaire design. Careful wording of a questionnaire (Box 36.3) is critical to a project's success.

3. Ensure that all those helping you with the study fully understand the protocol to be used. Whoever you involve in your study, make sure they fully understand its aims and objectives and exactly how the questionnaire is to be completed.

Motivate all those helping you with the project

You will inevitably have to rely on the goodwill and cooperation of many practice personnel to achieve a successful study; whether you need their help with handing out and collecting questionnaires, recruiting

Box 36.3   If you use a questionnaire to gather information for your project, be sure to design and word it carefully

1. Ensure that the questions are clear, easy to interpret and totally unambiguous
2. Wherever possible, pose questions that can be answered by circling a YES/NO or TRUE/FALSE option. Alternatively grade answers to a question from 1 to 5, and invite the patient to circle his or her response. If you use a grading system, it must be clearly defined; e.g. 5 = strongly agree, 4 = agree, 3 = neither agree nor disagree, 2 = disagree, 1 = strongly disagree
3. Avoid open-ended questions that invite an opinion or a view on an issue. It is difficult to analyse such subjective responses. In the HRT project, for example, do not ask patients why they have attended and leave a space for them to write their answer. Rather list a range of alternative answers for them to tick or circle. The options offered might include:

   I wish to protect my bones from thinning   ( )
   I wish to protect myself from heart disease   ( )
   I wish to relieve my symptoms of ......   ( )

   A patient could choose more than one option. One would not use as an option 'I wish to protect myself from osteoporosis' as this assumes that all patients are familiar with the term 'osteoporosis'. Questions must be user friendly, using terms that patients understand
4. Keep any questionnaire short. If it takes more than 5 minutes to complete, it will either not be completed or be completed inadequately, haphazardly or incorrectly
5. Run a brief pilot of your project with a few patients and adapt the wording of your questionnaire according to their comments

patients or collecting specimens, you will be heavily dependent on a range of staff. As well as being fully briefed on the study (including the starting date and the end-point), all those involved should be regularly updated on its progress and on any problems you are encountering. After the first few weeks the enthusiasm that you have engendered will wane—busy surgeries will have taken their toll, patients will be slipping through the net, MSUs will be going uncollected and questionnaires uncompleted or mislaid. Try and maintain the initial enthusiasm throughout the study. No simple project should last longer than 3 months, which is the maximum time you can realistically hope to maintain motivation.

The data collection stage

If your planning has been thorough, with all possible problems anticipated and avoided, data collection should be easy. Unfortunately you always have to expect the unexpected! Common problems and suggested solutions are listed in Table 36.1.

You must keep a daily watch on your project and how it is proceeding. The real enemy of project work is 'project drift'—the tendency for standards to drop and criteria to loosen as the project progresses. You must ensure that the last patient to enter your study is as rigorously assessed as the first.

The analysis and presentation stage

Once the data are collected, it is time for some quiet hours collating the results and analysing the questionnaires. It is too late to ask that extra question now! If you have chosen one or two simple questions and a YES/NO option for the answers, the results should be in the form of an easy to understand numerical list. If your data are to be fully appreciated, they must be presented properly. There are four main forms of data presentation: tables, graphs, pie diagrams and bar charts.

Tables

Do not try to cram all your results into one table; for clarity or presentation you may need three or four. Use clearly worded column headings, and give each table a clear caption that details what the table is designed to show.

Graphs

Graphs can show relationships very clearly but are rarely appropriate for a short, surgery-based project

Table 36.1 Common problems with data collection and suggested solutions

Problem	Suggested solution
Too few patients presenting with the condition	Should have been anticipated; encourage your team to be vigilant and recruit participants wherever possible
Poor cooperation from doctors and other staff on whose help the success of the study depends	Motivate your team throughout the project, not just at the start
Observer variation, either: within-observer variation (one observer recording differently at different times) or between-observer variation (different observers interpreting the interpretation project differently)	You should have standardized your methods of measurement or recording. Make it clear to all those participating what the precise criteria/methodology must be. There should be no room for individual variation
Inaccurate inclusions/exclusions to the study	Remind everyone recruiting patients of the entry criteria
Lost results/questionnaires	Chase them up! Keep a continual watch on the progress of your project
Improperly filled in questionnaires	Usually a result of poor design. You may be able to chase patients/doctors and persuade them to fill in the gaps

with only a handful of data. If you are using a graph, ensure that you make the best use of the space available, label your axes clearly and provide a detailed caption explaining what the graph is designed to demonstrate.

Bar charts or pie diagrams

Bar charts or pie diagrams (Fig. 36.1) are another effective way of presenting data visually. They work especially well when you wish to highlight a section of data.

Statistics

If your project is one of simple design that sets out to answer a practice-based question, the results are unlikely to need statistical analysis. With more ambitious research projects, however, such an analysis will be unavoidable.

As you move up the project ladder, and certainly if you wish critically to review other people's data, you will need to understand the fundamentals of statistics (Box 36.4).

Drawing conclusions

When you have tabulated your results, you will need to interpret their meaning. It is surprising how many research papers fall down at this stage. The authors may describe sound aims, objectives, methodology and data collection, yet draw the wrong conclusions.

The two broad errors to avoid when drawing conclusions are overgeneralization and failure to consider alternative explanations.

Do not overgeneralize

Your results will apply only to the precise population you have studied. If your study population of patients with cystitis consists of women aged 50–70 years, your results (and hence conclusions) will apply only to women aged 50–70 years. You might wish to extrapolate your results to the wider female population, but such comments will be entirely speculative; the situation among teenage girls may be totally different.

A major problem with small research projects is failure to obtain a representative random sample of the population studied. If you have only 20 patients in your study, you may by pure chance have two patients (i.e. 10%) who produce highly untypical results. These two freak values will skew the results significantly; whereas, if you had had 100 patients, two unusual results would have been diluted by the other 98 more 'normal' results. Small sample size will always make it difficult to draw meaningful conclusions.

Do not ignore alternative explanations

This is a real flaw in many project reports. When drawing conclusions from your results, you have to consider every possible explanation of the results. Supposing, for example, you find in the cystitis study

(a)

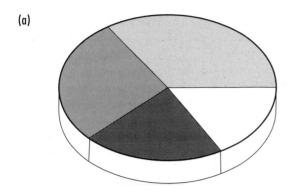

(b)

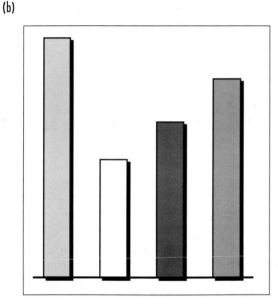

Fig. 36.1 A pie diagram (a) shows proportions much more clearly than a wordy explanation. Bar charts (b) are a good way of highlighting a particular section of data.

that positive MSUs were more common in January than in April. Considerations would have to be:

• Is the difference statistically significant? If 12 out of 20 patients had positive MSUs in January and 10 out of 20 had positive MSUs in April it is highly likely, in such a small sample with such a small difference, that these results could have occurred by chance—you have not demonstrated the supposed finding. If, however, 70 out of 100 patients had positive MSUs in January compared with 20 out of 100 in April, you might be on to something! 'You might

Box 36.4 Commonly used statistical terms

1. Mean: the sum of all the observations divided by the number of observations
2. Median: the observation in the middle; observations are arranged in a list, starting with the highest and ending with the lowest, and the observation in the middle is the median
3. Standard deviation: a measure of how sets of data are dispersed, i.e. how spread out the observations are. It gives a numerical measure of the variability of data. The commonly used measure is that of two standard deviations from the mean (mean +/− 2SD). This is the number which, when quoted, enables one to calculate between which two figures 95% of the observations fall. Take, for example, a study measuring the weight of patients. The mean might be expressed as 74 +/− 10 kg, the 10 kg being the 2 standard deviation from the mean. This means 95% of the weights fall between 64 and 84 kg. Put another way, 5% of the weights will fall outside these limits
4. P value: this is an important concept. If your results are truly going to demonstrate something, they must not have occurred by chance. The classic justification at the end of a results section is 'P < 0.05'. This means that the probability of these results having occurred by chance is less than 1 in 20 (i.e. less than 5%). By convention, P values of < 0.05 are termed statistically significant or, to be more precise, statistically significant at the 5% level; if P is < 0.5 for your results, the association you have demonstrated is likely to be valid. If your P value is > 0.05, it is entirely possible that chance could have generated your results and you can assume no association. If you obtain a P value of < 0.01, you can say that your results are highly statistically significant, there being a less than 1% probability that they have arisen by chance

be' is the correct way of describing it! You might not. There could be alternative explanations.

• Was your standardization right? Was there any project drift, with patients being accepted on strict criteria in January, whereas in April any patient with urinary frequency (even without dysuria) was included in the study to boost the numbers?

• Could the results be explained by some aspect of the specimen collection procedure? You might find that in April the collection system changed, so that MSUs were left for days before being processed and, as a result, fewer of them showed a significant growth.

The message is clear: before jumping to conclusions consider all the alternative explanations for your results.

Structure your discussion

If you are writing up a project, the discussion section should be structured in the following way:

• Discuss the actual results obtained, with refer-ence to the tables and figures constructed, in terms of what they show and what they do not show.

• Speculate about possible alternative explanations for the results.

• Discuss difficulties you encountered in under-taking the study and why they have biased the results; you may, for example, have inadvertently omitted a certain group of women from the study.

• Discuss the relevance of your results in terms of how they may alter your clinical practice.

• Suggest further studies that could answer ques-tions raised by the present project.

• Finally, try to relate the results of your study to those reported in the literature. Include references to related studies so that interested readers can widen their knowledge of the subject.

Acknowledgements
This chapter first appeared as an article in *Training Update* (February 1996) and is reproduced with per-mission from Reed Healthcare Communications Ltd.

37 MULTIPLE CHOICE QUESTIONS AND ANSWERS

1. Chapter 2

In a patient with glandular fever:

a. the Monospot test may take 2–3 weeks to turn positive
b. jaundice may occur in 5–10% of cases
c. a diagnosis can be made in practically all cases with clinical or laboratory means
d. a positive Monospot test is less likely in children than adults
e. tonsillectomy is indicated for severe cases.

2. Chapter 3

Advice to an acne sufferer would include:

a. avoidance of sunlight where possible
b. a strict low carbohydrate diet
c. wash at least twice a day with soap and water
d. squeeze the comedones (blackheads) prior to treatment
e. if on oral contraceptives use the more progestogenic variety.

3. Chapter 6

In an adult female patient presenting with uncomplicated cystitis:

a. she will have a 50% chance of significant bacteriuria in an MSU
b. oestrogen deficiency at the menopause is a recognized precipitating factor
c. a 7-day course of antibiotics should be given rather than a 3-day course
d. amoxycillin would be the antibiotic of first choice
e. trimethoprim would be the antibiotic of first choice.

4. Chapter 7

In tennis elbow:

a. there is localized tenderness on the medial side of the elbow
b. diagnosis can be made on X-ray
c. there is often restricted flexion at the elbow joint
d. injection therapy may initially exacerbate the pain
e. in most cases surgery is eventually necessary.

5. Chapter 8

In otitis media:

a. the inflammation starts in the pars flaccida of the drum
b. if antibiotics are indicated a 3-day course is sufficient
c. deafness is an important long-term complication
d. audiograms should be performed in all cases
e. Amoxycillin is the drug of choice in infants.

6. Chapter 9

In the general practice management of a patient with a myocardial infarction:

a. defibrillators are of limited use
b. the analgesic of choice is diamorphine
c. all patients should be given aspirin (unless a contraindication is known)
d. thrombolytic therapy is only of use in the first hour
e. most patients should be admitted to hospital.

7. Chapter 11

The following statements regarding the use of combined oral contraceptive preparations are correct:

a. with a pill starting on the first day of menstruation additional contraception is not required
b. it has a pregnancy rate of about 0.1–0.4 per 100 woman-years
c. if hypertension occurs it will always do so in the first year of use
d. it should be stopped if migraine appears for the first time
e. varicose veins are an absolute contraindication.

8. Chapter 12

The following are absolute contraindications to hormone replacement therapy:

a. an oestrogen dependent tumour
b. active thromboembolic disease
c. undiagnosed vaginal bleeding
d. severe active liver disease
e. smoking.

9. Chapter 13

With hay fever due to grass pollen:

a. it usually starts in July, ending in September
b. it may be regarded as a type I hypersensitivity
c. it is characterized by symptoms worse in the evening
d. desensitization should be carried out in the general practitioner's surgery for severely affected patients
e. inhaled steroids are more effective than inhaled cromoglycate in treating the allergic rhinitis.

10. Chapter 13

A stuffy nose may be caused by:

a. a nasal polyp
b. vasomotor rhinitis
c. house dust mite allergy
d. hay fever
e. prolonged use of vasoconstrictor decongestant.

11. Chapter 14

In depression:

a. tricyclic drugs can precipitate glaucoma
b. diurnal variation is a most useful predictive symptom
c. direct questions about suicidal intent should be avoided
d. anxiety is frequently an accompaniment
e. death of mother at any age makes the patient more likely to become depressed.

12. Chapter 15

In acute diarrhoea:

a. stool cultures yield 20% positive results
b. acute appendicitis is an important differential diagnosis

c. antibiotics are effective in half the cases
d. the presence of blood would be an indication for investigation
e. alcohol is rarely implicated.

13. Chapter 16

In scabies:

a. close bodily contact is needed for transmission
b. the best sites for burrows are between the fingers, the axillary folds and the anterior aspect of the wrist
c. there may be no initial itching
d. all family and contacts should be treated
e. secondary bacterial infection is uncommon.

14. Chapter 16

Ringworm

a. of the nails (tinea unguium) needs up to 4 weeks' treatment with terbinafine
b. of the foot (tinea pedis) may present as a severe vesicular form
c. of the groin (tinea cruris) can be spread by the sharing of sports clothes
d. of the groin (tinea cruris) responds well to topical steroid creams but frequently relapses
e. is most commonly diagnosed by culture on an agar plate.

15. Chapter 17

Characteristic features of acute glaucoma include:

a. a constricted pupil on the affected side
b. excessive discharge
c. normal visual acuity
d. severe pain in the affected eye
e. an association with ankylosing spondylitis.

16. Chapter 18

A patient presents to you with severe backache, sciatica and restriction of straight leg raising. You have diagnosed a slipped disc. The symptoms are:

a. likely to be aggravated by coughing
b. likely to be worse after rest
c. often recurrent
d. possibly serious if there are recent urinary symptoms present
e. best treated by laminectomy.

17. Chapter 19

The following patients should be targeted for screening for a raised serum cholesterol:

a. patients with existing heart disease
b. patients with hypertension
c. patients with diabetes
d. any patients with a corneal arcus
e. patients with a family history of hyperlipidaemia.

18. Chapter 20

With recurrent vaginal candidiasis:

a. use of antibiotics may be a predisposing factor
b. use of a vaginal diaphragm may be a predisposing factor
c. the patient should be advised to avoid nylon tights and pants
d. an exacerbation may occur in mid-cycle with ovulation
e. the urine should be tested for protein.

19. Chapter 21

A febrile convulsion may be classified as simple if it has the following characteristics:

a. it occurs in an infant
b. there are no local features
c. the fit lasts less than 15 minutes
d. there is a family history of febrile seizures
e. there are focal signs.

20. Chapter 22

The following are correlated with subsequent child abuse:

a. young parents
b. infrequent consultations at the doctor's surgery
c. premature birth
d. alcoholism
e. puerperal depression.

21. Chapter 23

Asthma:

a. affects about 1–2% of children
b. can present in childhood as a nocturnal cough
c. as a concept should rarely be discussed with patients
d. is usually overtreated by general practitioners
e. causes about 50 deaths a year in the UK.

22. Chapter 24

The following distinguishes croup from epiglottitis:

a. croup usually occurs in an older age group
b. the causative agent of croup is *Haemophilus influenzae*
c. dysphagia with drooling saliva is a typical symptom
d. there is usually a marked fever
e. there may be a loud stridor.

23. Chapter 25

Regarding the MMR vaccination:

a. the vaccine should be given at about 4 months of age
b. a history of fits is a contraindication
c. it is a live vaccine
d. a history of measles is a contraindication
e. the patient may develop a transient febrile illness about 8 days following immunization.

24. Chapter 26

The following statements are true of migraine:

a. it is in the first six of the most common causes of headache
b. it is a unilateral occipital pain
c. an attack lasts 4–72 hours
d. most patients have an aura preceding the headache
e. a family history is uncommon.

25. Chapter 28

In vertigo the following statements are true:

a. this symptom occurs twice as often in patients above the age of 65
b. a sensation of movement is crucial to the diagnosis
c. a negative Rinne test is diagnostic
d. the Valsalva manoeuvre is an effective remedy
e. it is frequently associated with wax in the ears.

26. Chapter 29

The following is true of dyslexia:

a. there is a marked tendency to be clumsy
b. girls are more often affected than boys
c. half those with reading retardation have this condition

d. there may be normal or superior spatial ability
e. a positive family history is strongly suggestive.

27. Chapter 30

When using morphine in the management of terminal illness:

a. it should be given on demand rather than regularly to prevent tolerance
b. doses of 100 mg or more are usually necessary
c. when injections are needed diamorphine is used
d. a phenothiazine is useful as an antiemetic
e. it should be used as a last resort due to its addictive properties.

28. Chapter 31

Simple napkin dermatitis (ammoniacal dermatitis):

a. is associated with infantile eczema
b. usually spares the skin creases
c. will be helped by waterproof plastic and rubber pants
d. can be improved by more frequent changing of nappies
e. should be treated with topical fluorinated steroids.

29. Chapter 33

With alcoholism:

a. most alcoholics will be known to their general practitioner
b. an average general practitioner will have about two alcoholics on his or her list
c. suicide is a definite risk
d. unexplained microcytosis in a blood film may be the first indication
e. research has demonstrated that there are marked differences between the available treatments.

30. All chapters

Screening in general practice is of proven benefit for:

a. cervical cancer
b. inflammatory bowel disease
c. hypertension
d. lung cancer
e. diabetes mellitus.

ANSWERS TO MULTIPLE CHOICE QUESTIONS

(True or False)

1. **Chapter 2**	aT	bT	cT	dT	eF
2. **Chapter 3**	aF	bF	cT	dF	eF
3. **Chapter 6**	aT	bT	cF	dF	eT
4. **Chapter 7**	aF	bF	cF	dT	eF
5. **Chapter 8**	aT	bT	cT	dF	eT
6. **Chapter 9**	aF	bT	cT	dF	eT
7. **Chapter 11**	aT	bT	cF	dT	eF
8. **Chapter 12**	aT	bT	cT	dT	eF
9. **Chapter 13**	aF	bT	cF	dF	eT
10. **Chapter 13**	aT	bT	cT	dT	eT
11. **Chapter 14**	aT	bT	cF	dT	eF
12. **Chapter 15**	aF	bT	cF	dT	eF
13. **Chapter 16**	aT	bT	cT	dT	eF
14. **Chapter 16**	aF	bT	cT	dF	eF
15. **Chapter 17**	aF	bF	cF	dT	eF
16. **Chapter 18**	aT	bF	cT	dT	eF
17. **Chapter 19**	aT	bT	cT	dF	eT
18. **Chapter 20**	aT	bF	cT	dF	eF
19. **Chapter 21**	aF	bT	cT	dF	eF
20. **Chapter 22**	aT	bF	cT	dT	eT
21. **Chapter 23**	aF	bT	cF	dF	eF
22. **Chapter 24**	aF	bF	cF	dF	eT
23. **Chapter 25**	aF	bF	cT	dF	eT
24. **Chapter 26**	aT	bF	cT	dF	eF
25. **Chapter 28**	aT	bT	cF	dF	eF
26. **Chapter 29**	aT	bF	cF	dT	eT
27. **Chapter 30**	aF	bF	cT	dT	eF
28. **Chapter 31**	aF	bT	cF	dT	eF
29. **Chapter 33**	aF	bF	cT	dF	eF
30. **All chapters**	aT	bF	cT	dF	eF

APPENDIX A

HAMILTON RATING SCALE (MODIFIED FOR SELF-RATING)

The assessment of depression has been greatly helped by the introduction of rating scales.

The Hamilton Rating Scale is shown here modified for self-administration. When it was tested in a clinical setting, depressed patients scored between 15 and 40, while controls scored less than 10.

The Beck Depression Inventory is commonly used also as a self-rating scale. It correlates well with an observer's rating. It indicates questions which are appropriate to the various aspects of depression (See Appendix B).

Q1
How depressed are you?
Score 0 If not at all
Score 1 If a little
Score 2 If moderately so
Score 3 If a lot
Score 4 If extremely so

Q2
Do you feel guilty about things that you have done or thought?
Score 0 If not at all
Score 1 If a little
Score 2 If moderately so
Score 3 If a lot
Score 4 If extremely so

Q3
Is it taking longer to get off to sleep?
Score 0 If not
Score 1 If sometimes
Score 2 If always

Q4
Do you sleep fitfully—often waking?
Score 0 If no

Score 1 If sometimes
Score 2 If always

Q5
Do you wake earlier than usual and then find yourself unable to get back to sleep?
Score 0 If no
Score 1 If sometimes
Score 2 If always

Q6
Have you lost interest in your work or hobbies?
Score 0 If not at all
Score 1 If a little
Score 2 If moderately so
Score 3 If a lot
Score 4 If extremely so

Q7
Is life pointless?
Score 0 If no
Score 1 If yes

Q8
Have you thought of ending it all?
Score 0 If no
Score 1 If yes

Q9
Have you made plans to kill yourself?
Score 0 If no
Score 1 If yes

Q10
Have you attempted to, or do you intend to, kill yourself?
Score 0 If no
Score 1 If yes

Q11
Do you feel that you are slower than your normal or usual speed?
Score 0 If not at all
Score 1 If a little
Score 2 If moderately so

Score 3 If a lot
Score 4 If extremely so

Q12

Do you feel anxious or tense?
Score 0 If not at all
Score 1 If a little
Score 2 If moderately so
Score 3 If a lot
Score 4 If extremely so

Q13

Do you suffer from any physical symptoms?
Score 0 If no
Score 1 If sometimes
Score 2 If always

Q14

Are you worried that you might have a serious illness such as cancer or VD
Score 0 If not at all
Score 1 If a little
Score 2 If moderately so
Score 3 If a lot
Score 4 If extremely so

Q15

Have you lost interest in sex?
Score 0 If not
Score 1 If sometimes
Score 2 If always

Q16

Have you lost weight recently—excluding that due to dieting?
Score 0 If no
Score 1 If yes—but clothes still fit
Score 2 If yes—but clothes now loose

Q17

Are you at your worst early in the day—but improve as the day goes on?
Score 0 If no
Score 1 If sometimes
Score 2 If always

Q18

Do you feel that either you or the outside world is unreal?
Score 0 If not at all
Score 1 If a little
Score 2 If moderately so
Score 3 If a lot
Score 4 If extremely so

(Source: Carr A C, Ancill R J, Ghosh A and Margo A 1981 Direct assessment of depression by microcomputer: a feasibility study. *Acta Psychiatr Scand* 64: 415–422.)

APPENDIX B

BECK DEPRESSION INVENTORY

A (Mood)
0 I do not feel sad
1 I feel blue or sad
2a I am blue or sad all the time and I can't snap out of it
2b I am so sad or unhappy that it is very painful
3 I am so sad or unhappy that I can't stand it

B (Pessimism)
0 I am not particularly pessimistic or discouraged about the future
1a I feel discouraged about the future
2a I feel I have nothing to look forward to
2b I feel that I won't ever get over my troubles
3 I feel that the future is hopeless and that things cannot improve

C (Sense of failure)
0 I do not feel like a failure
1 I feel I have failed more than the average person
2a I feel I have accomplished very little that is worth while or that means anything
2b As I look back on my life all I can see is a lot of failures
3 I feel I am a complete failure as a person (parent, husband, wife)

D (Lack of satisfaction)
0 I am not particularly dissatisfied
1a I feel bored most of the time
1b I don't enjoy things the way I used to
2 I don't get satisfaction out of anything any more
3 I am dissatisfied with everything

E (Guilty feelings)
0 I don't feel particularly guilty
1 I feel bad or unworthy a good part of the time
2a I feel quite guilty

2b I feel bad or unworthy practically all the time now
3 I feel as though I am very bad or worthless

F (Sense of punishment)
0 I don't feel I am being punished
1 I have a feeling that something bad may happen to me
2 I feel I am being punished or will be punished
3a I feel I deserve to be punished
3b I want to be punished

G (Self hate)
0 I don't feel disappointed in myself
1a I am disappointed in myself
1b I don't like myself
2 I am disgusted with myself
3 I hate myself

H (Self accusation)
0 I don't feel I am any worse than anybody else
1 I am very critical of myself for my weaknesses or mistakes
2a I blame myself for everything that goes wrong
2b I feel I have many bad faults

I (Self-punitive wishes)
0 I don't have any thoughts of harming myself
1 I have thoughts of harming myself but I would not carry them out
2a I feel I would be better off dead
2b I have definite plans about committing suicide
2c I feel my family would be better off if I were dead
3 I would kill myself if I could

J (Crying spells)
0 I don't cry any more than usual
1 I cry more now than I used to
2 I cry all the time now, I can't stop it
3 I used to be able to cry but now I can't cry at all even though I want to

K (Irritability)

0 I am no more irritated now than I ever am
1 I get annoyed or irritated more easily than I used to
2 I feel irritated all the time
3 I don't get irritated at all the things that used to irritate me

L (Social withdrawal)

0 I have not lost interest in other people
1 I am less interested in other people now than I used to be
2 I have lost most of my interest in other people and have little feeling for them
3 I have lost all my interest in other people and don't care about them at all

M (Indecisiveness)

0 I make decisions about as well as ever
1 I am less sure of myself now and try to put off making decisions
2 I can't make decisions any more without help
3 I can't make any decisions at all any more

N (Body image)

0 I don't feel I look any worse than I used to
1 I am worried that I am looking old or unattractive
2 I feel that there are permanent changes in my appearance and they make me look unattractive
3 I feel that I am ugly or repulsive looking

O (Work inhibition)

0 I can work about as well as before
1a It takes extra effort to get started at doing something
1b I don't work as well as I used to
2 I have to push myself very hard to do anything
3 I can't do any work at all

P (Sleep disturbance)

0 I can sleep as well as usual
1 I wake up more tired in the morning than I used to
2 I wake up 1–2 hours earlier than usual and find it hard to get back to sleep
3 I wake up early every day and can't get more than 5 hours' sleep

Q (Fatigability)

0 I don't get any more tired than usual
1 I get tired more easily than I used to
2 I get tired from doing anything
3 I get too tired to do anything

R (Loss of appetite)

0 My appetite is no worse than usual
1 My appetite is not as good as it used to be
2 My appetite is much worse now
3 I have no appetite at all any more

S (Weight loss)

0 I haven't lost much weight, if any, lately
1 I have lost more than 5 pounds (2.5 kilos)
2 I have lost more than 10 pounds (4.5 kilos)
3 I have lost more than 15 pounds (7 kilos)

T (Somatic preoccupation)

0 I am no more concerned about my health than usual
1 I am concerned about aches and pains or upset stomach or constipation or other unpleasant feelings in my body
2 I am so concerned with how I feel or what I feel that it's hard to think of much else
3 I am completely absorbed in what I feel

U (Loss of libido)

0 I have not noticed any recent change in my interest in sex
1 I am less interested in sex than I used to be
2 I am much less interested in sex now
3 I have lost interest in sex completely

(Source: Beck A T, Ward C H, Mendelson M, Mock J and Erbaugh J 1961 An inventory for measuring depression. *Arch Gen Psychiatry* 4:53).

APPENDIX C

ASSESSMENT OF CROHN'S DISEASE AND ULCERATIVE COLITIS (see Ch. 32)

This represents a numerically weighted scoring system which has been validated. It has been used internationally.

A score of >5 + has a high correlation with the subsequent diagnosis of Crohn's disease (86%), and a score of <5 + has a high correlation with the diagnosis of ulcerative colitis (Clamp SE et al *BMJ* 1982; 284: 91).

(It has not been used in the management of these conditions and it does not exclude intestinal tuberculosis.)

It is a useful check-list for monitoring the progress of these diseases and a changing score may well indicate a need for referral.

			Score
1. Age	1.1	<19	+1
	1.2	50–59	−1
	1.3	>70	−2
2. Family history	2.1	Ulcerative colitis	−2
	2.2	Crohn's disease	+4
3. Past history	3.1	Appendicitis	+3
	3.2	Anal fissure	+7
	3.3	Fistula	+4
	3.4	Nil	−1
4. Complications now present	4.1	Perianal	+7
	4.2	Fistula	+8
	4.3	Systemic	+1
	4.4	Nutrition emaciated	+2
5. Date of diagnosis	5.1	First consultation: use this section	
	5.2	1–3 months	−2
	5.3	3–6 months	−1
6. History of pain	6.1	Site Abdomen	
		6.1.1 Right lower quadrant	+10
		6.1.2 Left lower quadrant	−1
		6.1.3 Right half	+2
		6.1.4 Left half	−6
		6.1.5 Central	+2
		6.1.6 Nil	−1
	6.2	Type of pain	
		6.2.1 Severe	+2
		6.2.2 Steady	+2
7. Bowels	7.1	Frequency	
		7.1.1 Normal	+1
		7.1.2 × 1 day	+3
		7.1.3 × >10/day	−2
	7.2	Blood	
		7.2.1 Nil	+6
		7.2.2 Slight	−2
		7.2.3 ++	−5
	7.3	Mucus	
		7.3.1 Nil	+3
		7.3.2 Slight	−1
		7.3.3 ++	−2
8. Examination	8.1	Abdominal tenderness	
		8.1.1 Right lower quadrant	+10
		8.1.2 Upper half	−2
		8.1.3 Left half	−3
		8.1.4 Central	+6
		8.1.5 Nil	−1
	8.2	Distension	+2
	8.3	Mass	+10

INFLAMMATORY BOWEL DISEASE

Investigations used: radiology, endoscopy, biopsy, laboratory tests.

Radiology

Normal	−3
Continuous	−1
Segmental	+11

Site

Jejunum	+7
Ileum	+31
R Colon	+1
L Colon	−1
Rectum	−3

Findings

Stenosis	+4
Ulcers	−1

Dilatation	+4	Ulcers	−3
Fistula	+6	Giant cell	+20
Skip lesions	+8	Granuloma	+27
		Mucosal	−1
Endoscopy		Transmural	+16
Normal	+12		
Ulcers	−1	*Laboratory tests*	
Stenosis	+2	Hb < 10 g/dl	−1
Bleeding	−4	WCC > 20 000	+1
Diffuse	−2	Alb > 5 g/dl	−1
Patchy	+16	Plat > 150 000	−6
		> 400 000	+1
Biopsy		Iron 20–40	+1
Normal	+5		

(Data reproduced from Clamp S E, Myren J, Bouchier I A D, Watkinson G, De Dombal F T 1982 Diagnosis of inflammatory bowel disease: an international multicentre scoring system. *BMJ* 284:91, by permission of the authors and editor, *British Medical Journal*.)

INDEX